Type 2 Diabetes Diet Cookbook & Meal Plan:

55 Healthy Recipes for Diabetic People with an Easy 21 Day Meal Plan

ISBN-13: 978-1722340445
ISBN-10: 1722340444

Text copyright © 2018 Nigel Methews
All Rights Reserved.

Dedication

I dedicate this book to people who have to live with type 2 diabetes.

I very much wish that my book simplifies your life with diabetes, at least a little.. If the information in the book and the recipes will bring you at least a minute of joy - I deem that my goal has been achieved!

Content

Dedication 3

Introduction: 8

Chapter-1: All about Type-2 Diabetes 9

What is Type-2 Diabetes? 9

What are the causes of Type-2 Diabetes? 10

How does it affect the Body? 11

Chapter-2: Managing Diabetes 12

Chapter-3: Living the Anti-Diabetic Lifestyle: 15

Chapter-4: Best & Worst Foods for Diabetic Meal Plans 17

BREAKFAST RECIPES 22

Crustless Mushroom and Bok Choy Quiche 22

Scrambled Eggs with Sausage 25

Cheesy Mini Frittatas 27

Omelet-Topped Rosemary Veggies 29

Asparagus-Cheese Omelet 33

Spinach Frittata 36

Onion Tofu Scramble 38

Sausage Solo 40

Sausage Bacon Beans Cancan 42

Eggs Stuffed with Avocado & Watercress........44

LUNCH RECIPES 46

Chicken and Mushroom Stew 46

Lamb Stew 48

Spicy Whole Chicken..51

Bright Green Chicken Curry 53

Slow Cooker Mediterranean Stew....................56

Air Fried Chicken 58

Salmon Stew 60

Paprika Shrimp 62

Special Butter Fish 64

DINNER RECIPES 66

Harvested Chicken Stew..................................66

Shrimp Curry 68

Mexican Beef Brisket..70

Citrus Glazed Salmon 72

Beef Bulgogi 74

Delicious Lobster..76

Cheesy Cauliflower 78

Jamaican Jerk Pork Roast.......................................80

Pork Carnitas 82

SOUP RECIPES 84

Omega-3 Rich Salmon Soup 84

Cheesy Broccoli Soup 86

Egg Soup 88

Asparagus Soup 90

Chicken & Lime Soup 92

Beef & Veggies Soup 94

Salmon Soup 97

Ground Beef Soup 99

Shrimp Soup 101

DESSERTS RECIPES..103

Berries and Cream..103

Fresh Strawberry Granita 105

Limeabalemon Glaciate 107

Crème Brûlée...109

Pumpkin Custard..111

Thai Coconut Custard......................................113

Chocolate Peanut Butter Cups 115

Cream Crepes 117

Nut Porridge 119

BAKERY PRODUCTS RECIPES 121

Flourless Chocolate Brownies 121

Spinach Quiche 123

Peanut Butter Cookies 125

Cheddar Biscuits 127

Cheesecake Cupcakes 129

Sausage Waffles 131

Peach Muffins 133

Simple Savory Bread 136

Chocolate Cheese Cake 139

21 Days Meal Plan 141

CONCLUSION: 146

Legal Notice 147

Introduction:

Diabetes is the fastest growing disease in the USA. In 2015, 392 million people across the globe had this disease. It shortens your life expectancy by a decade and is very rapidly growing in youngsters. It can be easily prevented by having a proper and healthy diet plan, exercising regularly with a proper routine, and maintaining a feasible weight according to your height.

Chapter-1: All about Type-2 Diabetes

What is Type-2 Diabetes?

It is a medical condition in which the blood sugar level (glucose) rises above the allowed limit or its normal value. It is also known as 'hyperglycemia'. In this condition, the body doesn't utilize the insulin present in the body, and this is known as insulin resistance. In the beginning stages, the pancreas starts dealing with the issue and tends to produce sufficient insulin; but with time, this process slows down, and there is not insulin present to normalize blood sugar levels in the body.

Type-2 diabetes is also referred to as a long term metabolic disorder in which there is lack of insulin, higher blood sugar levels, and insulin resistance. The most common symptoms of type2 diabetes include excessive urination, increase in thirstiness; pain or tingling in the legs, feet, or hands; and sudden weight loss. Other symptoms may include tiredness, increase in hunger, and lower healing capabilities for injuries/sores. The symptoms of this disease show slowly with time and aren't instantly visible, making it hard to diagnose without the proper tests. There are various long-term effects of diabetes, like cardiac arrests and strokes, diabetic retinopathy (which leads to blindness), kidney failure, and improper flow of blood leading to amputation of certain body parts. The uncommon effect of this disease is ketoacidosis which might lead to coma and eventually death.

What are the causes of Type-2 Diabetes?

There are various causes of type-2 diabetes and more than a single factor is involved in creating this disease. The most common cause of type-2 diabetes is a history of this disease in the family, making it more like a genetic prone disease. Having all or any of these causes will increase your risk of having type-2 diabetes. Some of them include:

1. Poor diet management.
2. Being obese and overweight.
3. Increasing age factor.
4. High blood pressure and cholesterol levels.
5. No control of blood glucose.
6. Living a sedentary lifestyle.
7. Illnesses or pregnancy.

Many studies are being conducted to pinpoint the causes of type-2 diabetes due to the increasing number of its patients. A genetic issue is still considered to be the most popular cause of this disease, as certain genes increase the likelihood of developing of type-2 diabetes. This disease is found more in ethnicities having ancestors of Middle Eastern, African-Caribbean, and South Asian origins. Another important factor for the cause of type-2 diabetes is diet, but there is always a debate in the scientific and medical corners about which specific diets or parts of it are to be held responsible for this metabolic disorder. Despite the debate, processed foods, higher carb intake, and saturated & trans fats are credited as the reason for developing type-2 diabetes.

How does it affect the Body?

1. Results in coronary heart disease.
2. Raises blood pressure and cholesterol levels, which results in heart attacks and cardiovascular complications.
3. Causes strokes.
4. Diabetic retinopathy.
5. Causes diabetic nephropathy (a kidney disease).
6. Tingling, numbness or pain in the hands, legs and feet.
7. Sexual dysfunction.
8. Increased sweating.
9. Frequent urination and increased thirst.
10. Can also cause diarrhea, constipation, and nausea.
11. Can cause skin issues, like slower healing capacity of wounds, injuries, sores, bacterial and fungal infections, burns and cuts in addition to loss of feelings or numbness in the feet.

Chapter-2: Managing Diabetes

Changing Your Outlook:

Living with diabetes is not as hard as it is portrayed, but it does need a lot of will power. Diabetes is directly linked with obesity, which means that to remain healthy, you have to transform your physical physique into the required one. It requires you to lose that extra weight you put on through regularly exercising outside of food changes. Working out might not be that easy with diabetes as you feel increased thirst, tingling, and many other physical symptoms which are going to make losing weight very hard for you. But weight loss is going to make your life much easier and might even lower the impacts of diabetes on your body.

Transforming Your Lifestyle:

Being diabetic requires certain stern changes in your lifestyle, which are critically important to deal with your disease in an effective manner and avoid any further complications or worsening of the disease itself. Some important factors which you have to be concerned about while managing a diabetic life are as follows:

Food:
1. Understand carb count and its portion sizes.
2. Devise a balanced meal plan and follow it.
3. Have coordination between your medicines and meals.
4. Never ever go for beverages contain sugar sweeteners like soda, etc.

Workout Sessions:
1. Consult your doctor for an expert's opinion for devising an exercise plan.
2. Keep a properly devised exercise routine and maintain it.
3. Regularly check your health-related levels like sugar, insulin, cholesterol, etc.
4. Have a strict check on your blood sugar levels.
5. Drink enough water.
6. Make adjustments in your treatment plan for diabetes whenever required and needed.

Medication:
1. Have a proper storage for your insulin.
2. Always see your general physician anything happens irrespective of your nature.
3. Consider taking precautionary steps while trying new medications.

Illness:
1. Thoroughly plan out your treatment plan.
2. Don't cease your diabetes related medications.
3. Strictly follow your diabetic meal plans.

Alcohol:
1. Consult your doctor for his opinion on alcohol consumption.
2. Never consume alcohol while being on an empty stomach.
3. Always opt for drinks with care.
4. Have a count of your caloric intake regularly.
5. Note your blood glucose/sugar levels prior to going to bed.

Menstruation and menopause:
1. Note down your patterns and keep them in mind.
2. Make necessary adjustments in your diabetes meal plan accordingly.
3. Frequently note your blood sugar levels.

Stress:
1. Understand your stress
2. Take control of the situation.
3. Seek help whenever felt the need for.

Chapter-3: Living the Anti-Diabetic Lifestyle:

Scrutinizing Your Meals:

Maintain a proper diet plan, keep it balanced, and use alternative meals for various foods to avoid any further worsening of your disease. Create a proper nutritious diet with knowledge of your carb intake and your portion sizes, etc. Never ever go for sodas and other sugar sweetened drinks. Keep yourself from sugar to have a convenient lifestyle with diabetes.

Tracking Your Physical Activity:

Diabetes is directly linked to obesity, so you must maintain a proper weight and remain under a certain level. To accomplish this, you have to do physical activities, like work out sessions, jogging, and other activities. Before devising an exercise plan, do consult your doctor for his expert opinion and devise a plan according to his suggestions and then strictly follow that plan. No matter how you work out, REMAIN HYDRATED! Diabetics have increased thirst and excessive sweating, so you must drink adequate water to overcome that and remain fit. Also note your health factors, like blood sugar level, blood pressure levels, and cholesterol levels.

Planning Your Next Meal:

Plan your meals with a strict anti-diabetes meal plan and stick to it no matter what. Your food plays an important factor in managing your diabetic lifestyle. Consult your doctor for suggestions, and efficiently follow the diet plan to avoid any worsening of the disease.

Diet Alternatives:

There are various diet alternatives available for sugar added foods. You can easily get these alternatives at various stores and pharmacies.

Chapter-4: Best & Worst Foods for Diabetic Meal Plans

GRAINS:
ALLOWED:
1. Oats
2. Quinoa

NOT ALLOWED:
1. Pastries
2. White Bread

PROTEINS:
ALLOWED:
1. Beans & Lentils
2. Wild Salmon
3. Greek Yogurt

NOT ALLOWED:
1. Char-Grilled Meat
2. Country Fried Steak

VEGGIES AND FRUITS:
ALLOWED:
1. Leafy Greens
2. Cruciferous Vegetables
3. Berries

NOT ALLOWED:
1. Fries
2. Fruit Smoothies

FATS:

ALLOWED:
1. Avocado
2. Chia Seeds
3. Raw Almonds
4. Ground Flaxseeds

NOT ALLOWED:
1. Roasted Nuts
2. Shortening

DRINKS:

ALLOWED:
1. Green Tea
2. Coffee

NOT ALLOWED:
1. Sports Drinks
2. Soda
3. Fancy Coffee Drinks

Glycemic Index for foods: (The entire data is average ± SEM.)

Food	Glycemic Index (Glucose= 100)	Foods	Glycemic Index (Glucose= 100)
Snacks		**Legumes**	
Popcorn	65±5	Kidney Beans	24±4
Chocolates	40±3	Soya Beans	16±1
Potato Crisps	56±3	Chick Peas	28±9
Rice Crackers/Crisps	87±2	Lentils	32±5
Soda/Soft Drinks	59±3	**Sugars**	
Fruits & Fruit Products		Honey	61±3
Orange Juice	50±2	Sucrose	65±4
Apple Juice	41±2	Fructose	15±4
Pineapple, Raw	59±8	Glucose	103±3
Water Melon, Raw	76±4	**Veggies**	
Strawberry Jam/Jelly	49±3	Potato, Fries	63±5

Mango, Raw†	51±5	Potato, mashed	87±3
Apple, Raw†	36±2	Potato, boiled	78±4
Banana, Raw†	51±3	Sweet Potato. Boiled	63±6
Orange, Raw†	43±3	Pumpkin, Boiled	64±7
Peach, Canned†	43±5	Taro, Boiled	53±2
Dates, Raw	42±4	Carrots, Boiled	39±4
Dairy Products		Green banana/ Plantain	55±6
Skimmed Milk	37±4	Vegetable Soup	48±5
Full Fat Milk	39±3	**High Carb Foods**	
Fruit Yogurt	41±2	Chapatti	52±4
Rice Milk	86±7	Specialty Grain Bread	53±2
Ice Cream	51±3	Wheat Roti	62±3
Soy Milk	34±4	Corn Tortilla	46±4
Breakfast Cereals		Barley	28±2
Rolled Oats Porridge	55±2	White Spaghetti	49±2
Porridge, Instant Oat	79±3	Boiled White Rice*	73±4

Millet Porridge	67±5	White wheat Bread*	75±2
Cornflakes	81±6	Boiled Brown Rice	68±4
Congee/ Rice Porridge	78±9	Sweet Corn	52±5
Muesli	57±2	Rice Noodles†	53±7
Wheat Flakes Biscuits	69±2	Couscous†	65±4

'†' Varieties with lower GI are also included.

'*' Mean value of all the available data.

BREAKFAST RECIPES

Crustless Mushroom and Bok Choy Quiche

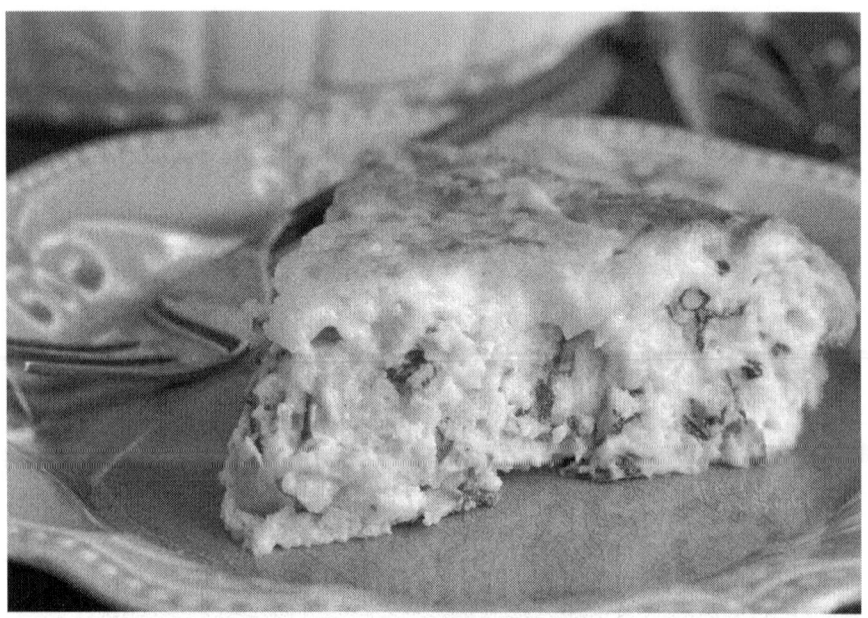

Ingredients:

- 2 tablespoons olive oil
- ¼ teaspoon freshly ground black pepper
- 2 onions, chopped
- 1 cup Portobello mushrooms, coarsely chopped
- 10 eggs, beaten
- 6 cups Swiss cheese, shredded
- ½ teaspoon salt
- 1 (10 ounce) package Bok Choy, thawed and drained

How to prepare:

1. Preheat your oven to 350F.
2. Grease a pie pan with cooking spray.
3. Sauté onion in heated oil in a large wok for about 3 minutes and add Bok Choy.
4. Cook for 3 more minutes until the excess moisture has evaporated.
5. Whisk together eggs, cheese, salt and black pepper in a large bowl.
6. Transfer the egg mixture and Bok Choy mixture in an immersion blender and blend until smooth.
7. Transfer the blended mixture into prepared pie pan and place the pan in the oven.
8. Bake for 18 minutes.

Preparation time: 20 minutes

Cooking time: 24 minutes

Total time: 46 minutes

Servings: 12

Nutritional Values:

Calories 155

Total Fat 11.2 g

Saturated Fat 5.1 g

Cholesterol 151 mg

Sodium 235 mg

Total Carbs 4.1 g

Fiber 1.4 g

Sugar 1.6 g

Protein 10.5 g

Potassium 347 mg

Scrambled Eggs with Sausage

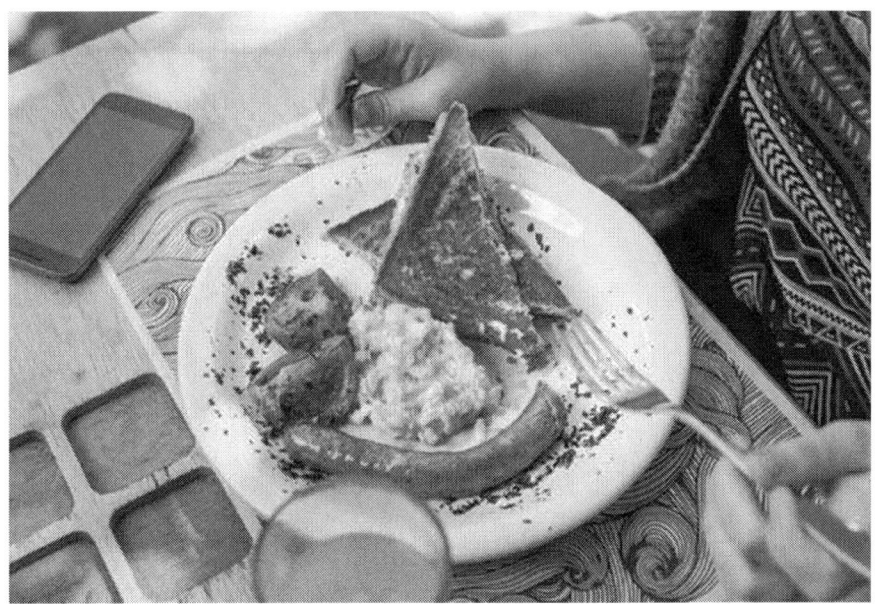

Ingredients:

- 2 ounce cooked turkey sausage, sliced
- 4 eggs
- 4 tablespoons reduced-sodium chicken broth
- 4 tablespoons reduced-fat cheddar cheese, finely shredded
- Pinch ground black pepper
- ½ cup cherry tomatoes, quartered

How to prepare:
1. Preheat the skillet over medium heat and coat it with a cooking spray.
2. Whisk together broth, eggs, and black pepper in a medium bowl and add sliced sausages.

3. Pour this mixture into hot skillet and cook over medium heat until the mixture begins to set on the bottom and around edges.
4. Lift and fold the incompletely cooked egg mixture with a large spatula so that the uncooked portion flows beneath.
5. Add tomatoes and cheese and cook for about 1 minute until egg mixture is cooked through.
6. Dish out in a serving plate and serve hot.

Preparation time: 10 minutes
Cooking time: 10 minutes
Total time: 20 minutes
Servings: 4

Nutritional Values:
Calories 146
Total Fat 10.9 g
Saturated Fat 4.2 g
Cholesterol 183 mg
Sodium 260 mg
Total Carbs 1.4 g
Fiber 0.3 g
Sugar 1 g
Protein 10.6 g
Potassium 174 mg

Cheesy Mini Frittatas

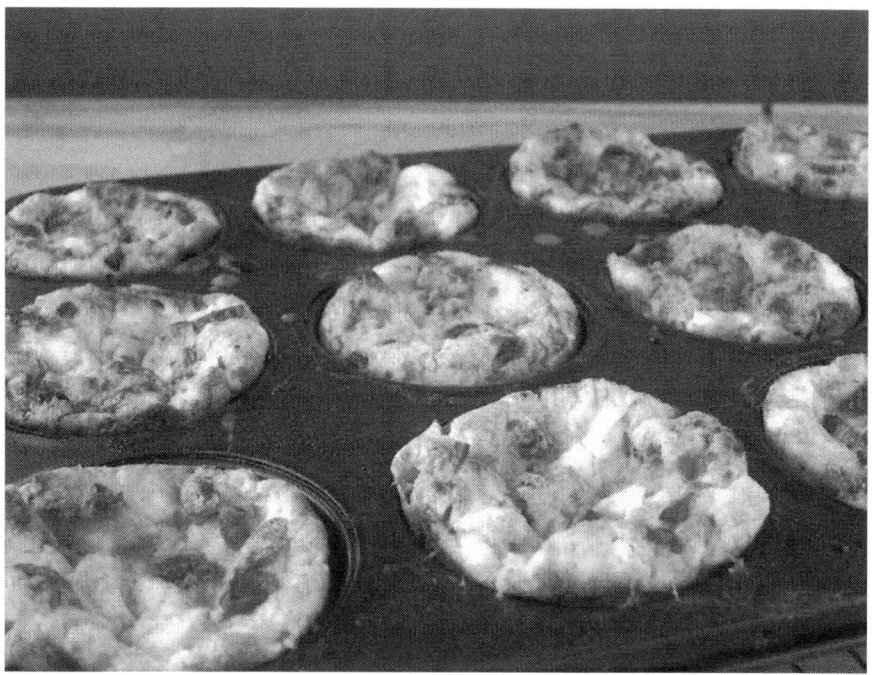

Ingredients:

- 6 organic eggs
- 8 tablespoons cheddar cheese, shredded
- 2 scallions, chopped
- ½ cup unsweetened almond milk
- ½ teaspoon lemon pepper seasoning
- 4 cooked bacon slices, crumbled
- 2 medium zucchini, finely chopped
- ½ teaspoon, or to taste, salt and black pepper

How to prepare:
1. Preheat your oven to 325F and spray the silicone molds with cooking spray.
2. Combine all the ingredients in a bowl using an electric beater and transfer the mixture into silicone molds.
3. Place the molds inside the oven and bake for about 20 minutes.
4. Remove from the oven and serve immediately.

Preparation time: 10 minutes
Cooking time: 20 minutes
Total time: 30 minutes
Servings: 6

Nutritional Values:

Calories 185

Total Fat 13.2 g

Saturated Fat 5.1 g

Cholesterol 188 mg

Sodium 435 mg

Total Carbs 3.5 g

Fiber 1 g

Sugar 1.6 g

Protein 13.6 g

Omelet-Topped Rosemary Veggies

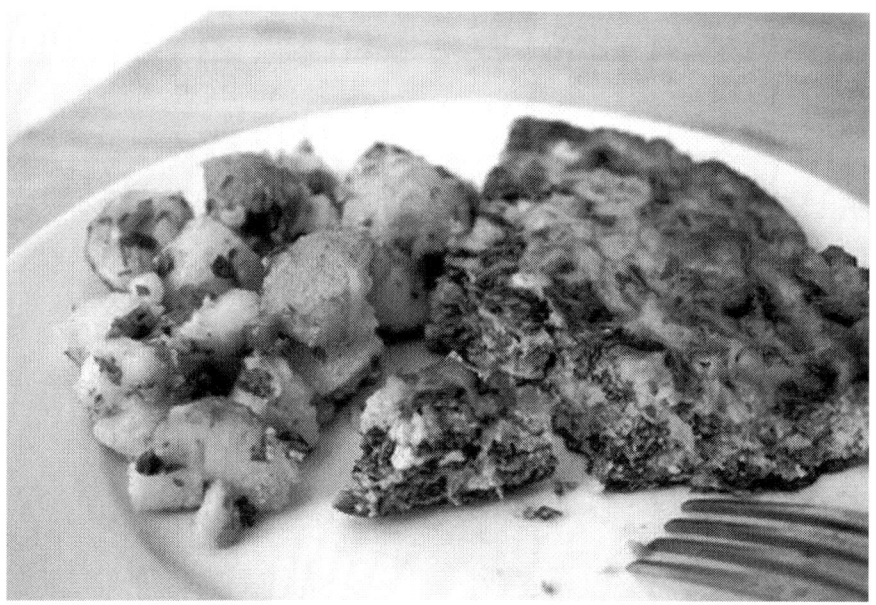

Ingredients:

- 4 tablespoons water
- 2 (12-ounce) package frozen and roasted red potatoes and green beans with rosemary butter sauce
- Non-stick cooking spray
- 6 tablespoons fresh chives, snipped
- 6 eggs
- ½ cup cheddar cheese, reduced fat

How to prepare:

1. Microwave the vegetables and coat a large nonstick skillet lightly with a cooking spray.
2. Preheat the skillet over medium-high heat and whisk together egg and water in a bowl.
3. Add this mixture into the skillet and cook over medium-high heat for 2 minutes, without stirring.
4. Lift the egg mixture so that the uncooked portion flows beneath.
5. Cook a minute more or until the egg mixture is just set.
6. Turn over the omelet and turn off heat.
7. Add the vegetables to a pie plate of 9-inch and top with omelet.
8. Fold the edges to fit dish and sprinkle with cheddar cheese.
9. Heat in a microwave oven for about 30 seconds until the cheese is melted.
10. Top with chives and dish out to serve hot

Preparation time: 20 minutes
Cooking time: 30 minutes
Total time: 50 minutes
Servings: 6

Nutritional Values:

Calories 155

Total Fat 11.2 g

Saturated Fat 5.1 g

Cholesterol 151 mg

Sodium 235 mg

Total Carbs 4.1 g

Fiber 1.4 g

Sugar 1.6 g

Protein 10.5 g

Potassium 347 mg

Asparagus-Cheese Omelet

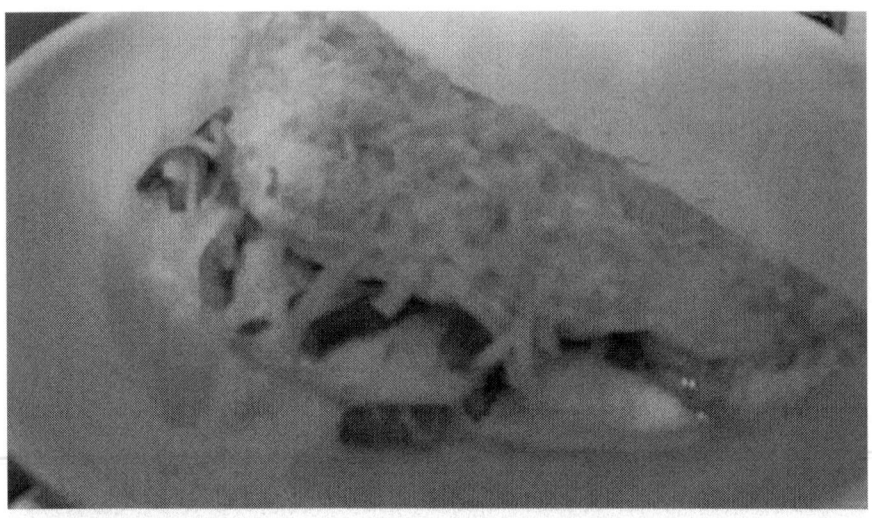

Ingredients:

- 2 teaspoons olive oil
- 12 thin asparagus spears
- 4 ounce desired flavor individually foil-wrapped spreadable cheese wedge, cut up
- 12 egg whites
- 4 tablespoons red bell pepper slivers
- 1 teaspoon freshly ground black pepper
- 4 teaspoons fresh parsley, snipped

How to prepare:

1. Grease a nonstick skillet using a cooking spray and add asparagus.

2. Cook for 7 minutes over medium-high heat, occasionally rotating.
3. Cover with foil and keep aside.
4. Mix together red bell pepper and egg whites in a bowl.
5. Mix well until combined with the help of a fork, but do not make it frothy.
6. Heat oil in the skillet and add egg whites.
7. Lower the heat to medium and gently lift edges of set egg white with a spatula.
8. Lean the pan so that the liquid egg white runs under the set egg.
9. Repeat it until the egg is set but still shiny.
10. Place the asparagus spears on half of the eggs in skillet and evenly sprinkle with cheese.
11. Make half-moon omelet by overlapping half of the eggs over the cheese and asparagus.
12. Dish out the omelet and top with red bell pepper slivers and parsley.

Preparation time: 10 minutes
Cooking time: 10 minutes
Total time: 20 minutes
Servings: 4

Nutritional Values:

Calories 116

Total Fat 5 g

Saturated Fat 1 g

Cholesterol 10 mg

Sodium 427 mg

Total Carbs 4 g

Fiber 1 g

Sugar 3 g

Protein 15 g

Potassium 356 mg

Spinach Frittata

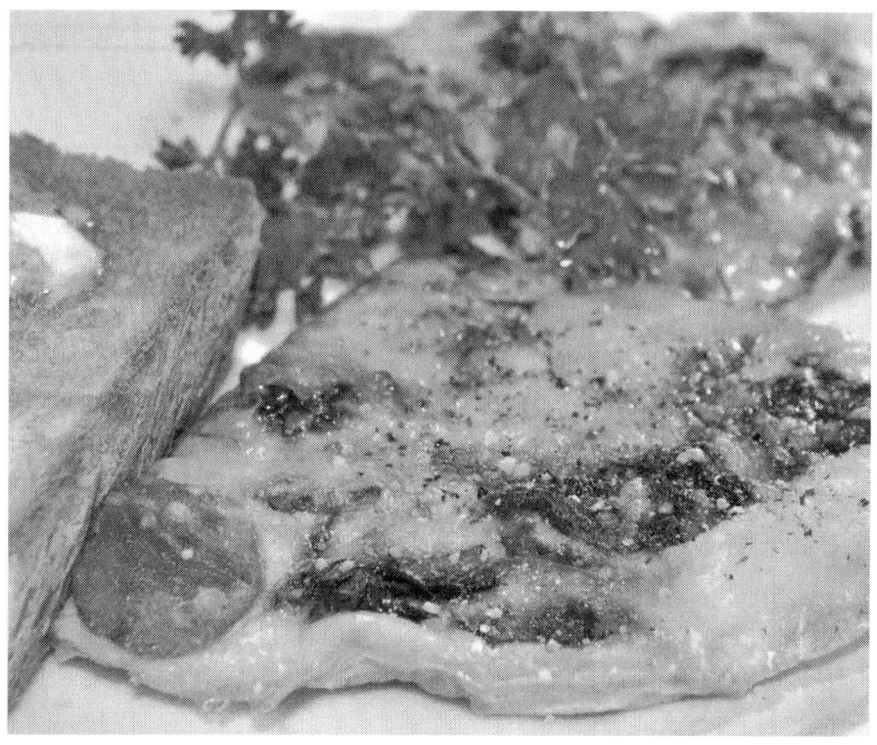

Ingredients:

- 3 organic egg whites
- ½ cup onions, chopped
- 1 cup fresh spinach, chopped
- 2 tablespoons fat-free milk
- 1 cup low-fat mozzarella cheese, shredded and divided
- 2 organic eggs
- 1 tablespoon olive oil
- 1 medium tomato, chopped

- 1 garlic clove, minced
- ¼ teaspoon sea salt and pepper

How to prepare:
1. In a bowl, whisk eggs and milk and keep aside.
2. Heat the olive oil in a skillet and add garlic and onions.
3. Sauté for about 4 minutes and add whisked eggs.
4. Sauté for about 2 minutes and add the remaining ingredients.
5. Cook covered for about 15 minutes.
6. Dish out and serve hot.

Preparation time: 10 minutes
Cooking time: 21 minutes
Total time: 31 minutes
Servings: 3

Nutritional Values:
Calories 153
Total Fat 10 g
Saturated Fat 2.8 g
Cholesterol 143 mg
Sodium 154 mg
Total Carbs 5.3 g
Fiber 1.1 g
Sugar 3 g
Protein 11.2 g
Potassium 117 mg

Onion Tofu Scramble

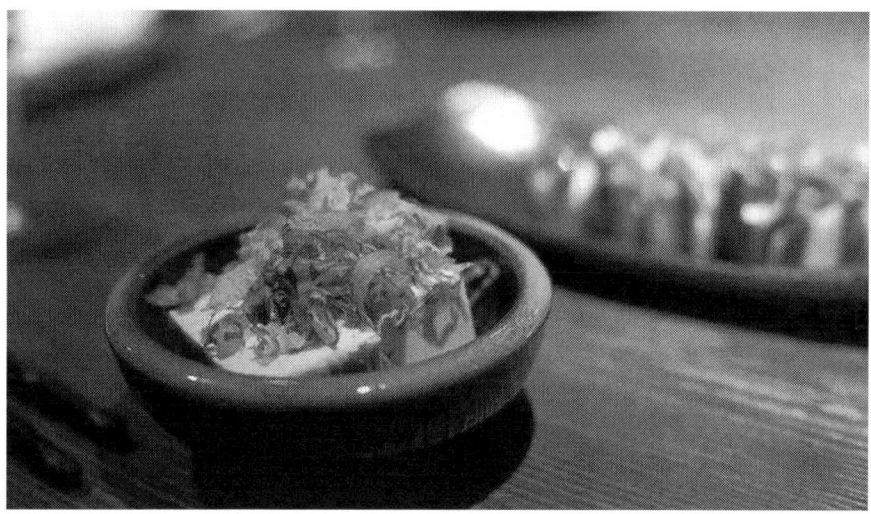

Ingredients:

- 4 medium onions, sliced
- 2 cups cheddar cheese, grated
- 4 blocks tofu, pressed and cubed into 1 inch pieces
- 4 tablespoons butter
- ¼ teaspoon salt and freshly ground black pepper

How to prepare:

1. Mix together tofu, salt, and black pepper in a bowl and keep aside.
2. Melt butter in a pan and add onions.
3. Cook for about 3 minutes and add tofu mixture.
4. Cook for about 2 minutes and add cheddar cheese.

5. Cook covered for 6 minutes on low.
6. Dish out and serve hot.

Preparation time: 8 minutes
Cooking time: 13 minutes
Total time: 20 minutes
Servings: 6

Nutritional Values:

Calories 184

Total Fat 12.7 g

Saturated Fat 7.3 g

Cholesterol 35 mg

Total Carbs 6.3 g

Sugar 2.7 g

Fiber 1.6 g

Sodium 222 mg

Potassium 174 mg

Protein 12.2 g

Sausage Solo

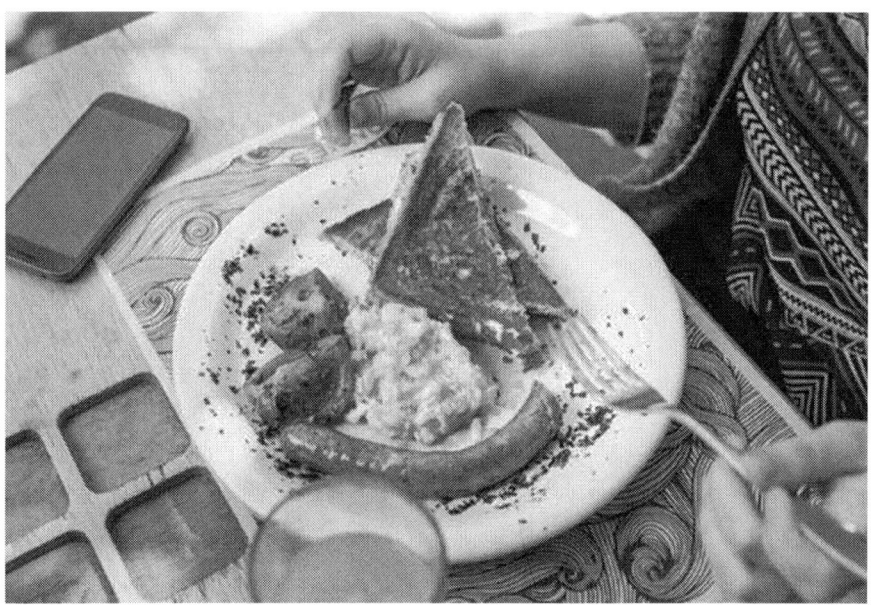

Ingredients:

- 2 eggs
- ¼ cup cream
- 2 cooked sausages, sliced
- 1 tablespoon butter
- ¼ cup mozzarella cheese, grated

How to prepare:
1. Preheat your oven to 360 F and grease 2 ramekins with butter.
2. Whisk together eggs and cream in a bowl and transfer the egg mixture into ramekins.

3. Top evenly with sausage slices and cheese and place ramekins in the oven.
4. Bake for about 20 minutes and immediately serve.

Preparation time: 5 minutes
Cooking time: 30 minutes
Total time: 35 minutes
Servings: 2

Nutritional Values:

Calories 180
Total Fat 12.7 g
Saturated Fat 4.7 g
Cholesterol 264 mg
Total Carbs 3.9 g
Sugar 1.3 g
Fiber 0.1 g
Sodium 251 mg
Potassium 142 mg
Protein 12.4 g

Sausage Bacon Beans Cancan

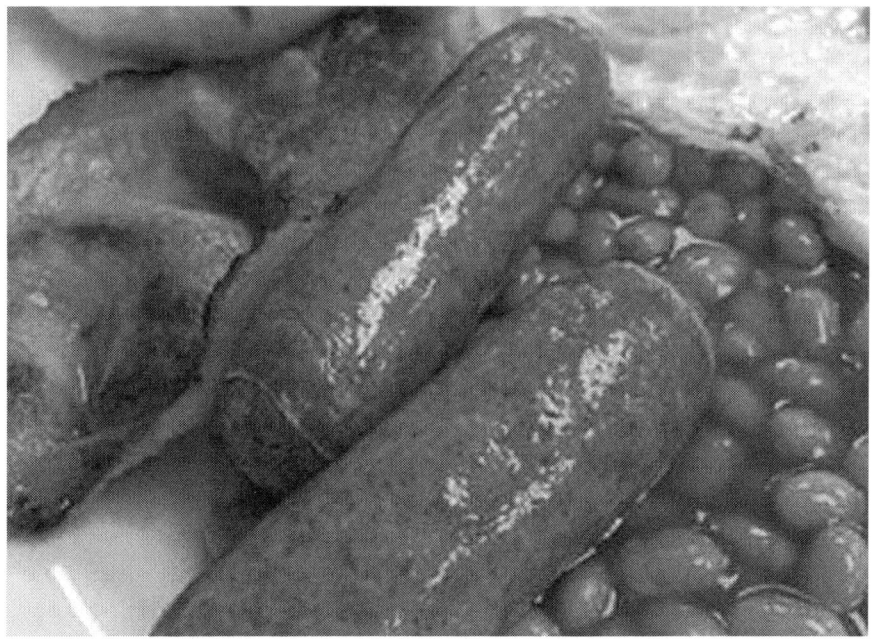

Ingredients:

- 3 bacon slices
- ½ tablespoon butter
- 3 medium sausages
- ¼ can white beans, boiled
- 1/8 teaspoon salt and pepper

How to prepare:
1. Season the sausages with salt and black pepper.
2. Heat the butter in the skillet and add sausages.
3. Cook for about 3 minutes and stir in beans and bacon slices.

4. Cover the lid and let simmer for 4 minutes on low heat.
5. Dish out and serve immediately.

Preparation time: 8 minutes
Cooking time: 7 minutes
Total time: 15 minutes
Servings: 3

Nutritional Values:
Calories 199
Total Fat 12 g
Saturated Fat 4 g
Cholesterol 32 mg
Total Carbs 9.5 g
Sugar 0.3 g
Fiber 2.3 g
Sodium 538 mg
Potassium 354 mg
Protein 13 g

Eggs Stuffed with Avocado & Watercress

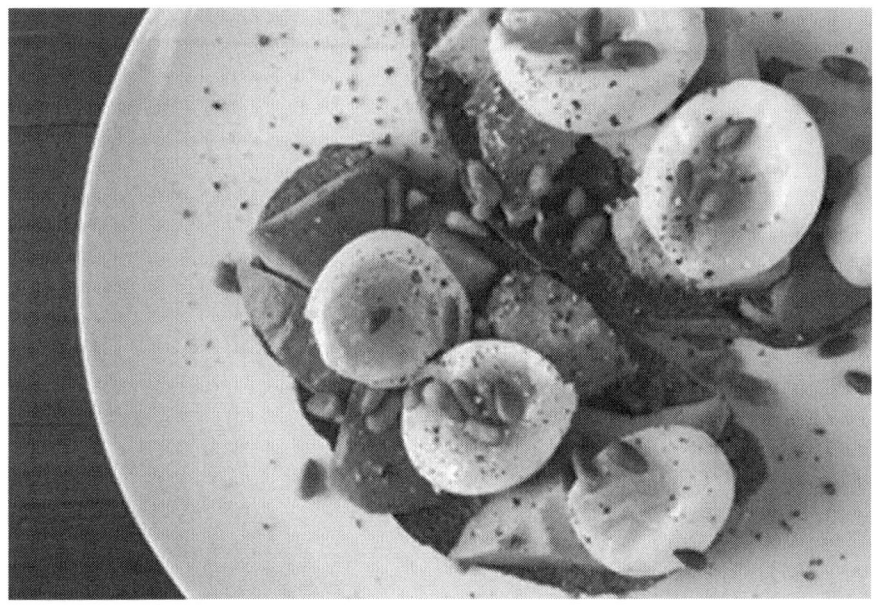

Ingredients:

- ½ medium ripe avocado, peeled, pitted, and chopped
- ¼ tablespoon fresh lemon juice
- 3 organic eggs, boiled, peeled, and cut in half lengthwise
- ¼ cup fresh watercress, trimmed
- Salt, to taste

How to prepare:
1. Arrange a trivet at the bottom of an Instant Pot and add water.
2. Put the watercress on the trivet and secure the lid.

3. Press the "Manual" button and cook at high pressure for about 3 minutes.
4. Quickly release the pressure and drain the watercress completely.
5. Remove the egg yolks and transfer into a bowl.
6. Add watercress, avocado, salt and lemon juice and mash with a fork.
7. Arrange the egg whites in a serving plate and stuff with watercress mixture.

Preparation time: 10 minutes
Cooking time: 5 minutes
Total time: 15 minutes
Servings: 3

Nutritional Values:
Calories 132
Total Fat 10.9 g
Saturated Fat 2.7 g
Cholesterol 164 mg
Total Carbs 3.3 g
Sugar 0.5 g
Fiber 2.3 g
Sodium 65 mg
Potassium 226 mg
Protein 6.3 g

LUNCH RECIPES

Chicken and Mushroom Stew

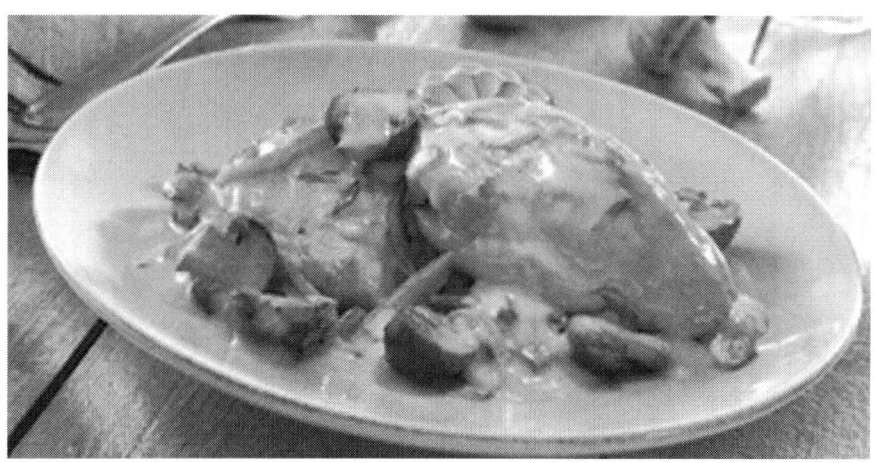

Ingredients:

- 1 small onion, chopped
- 2 cup fresh cherry tomatoes
- 1 cup fresh parsley, chopped
- 1 cup green olives, pitted and halved
- 8 (2.5-ounce) skinless chicken thighs
- 1 pound fresh cremini mushrooms, stemmed and quartered
- 2 garlic cloves, minced
- ½ cup low-sodium chicken broth
- 1 tablespoon olive oil
- 1 tablespoon tomato paste
- Freshly ground black pepper, to taste

How to prepare:

1. Sauté the onions and mushrooms for about 5 minutes in heated oil and add garlic and tomato paste.
2. Cook for about 1 minute and stir in the chicken, olives, tomatoes, and chicken broth.
3. Cook covered for 18 minutes on medium-low heat.
4. Stir in parsley and black pepper and dish out to serve.

Preparation time: 5 minutes
Cooking time: 26 minutes
Total time: 31 minutes
Servings: 6

Nutritional Values:

Calories 238

Total Fat 9.7 g

Saturated Fat 2.3 g

Cholesterol 84 mg

Sodium 112 mg

Total Carbs 6.5 g

Fiber 1.5 g

Sugar 2.7 g

Protein 30.2 g

Potassium 716 mg

Lamb Stew

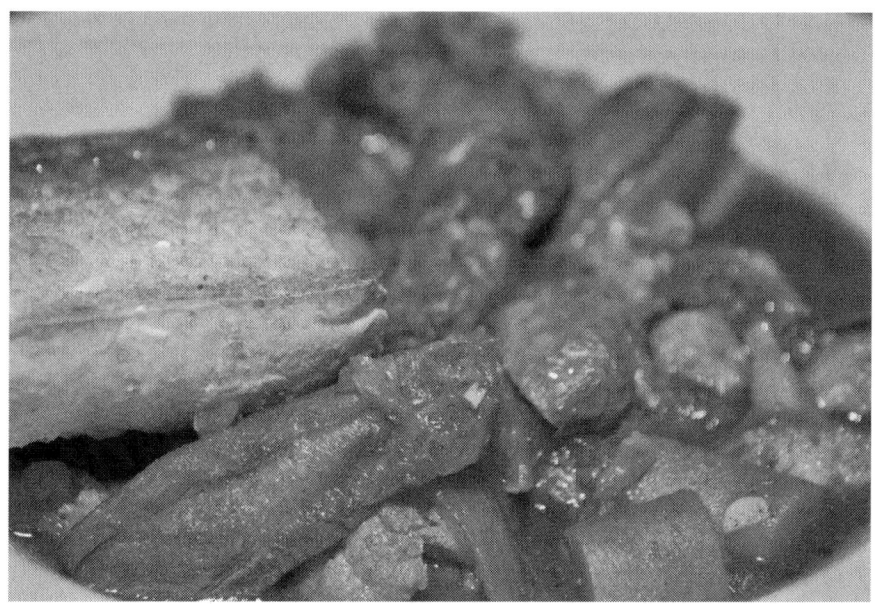

Ingredients:

- ½ small yellow onion, chopped
- 1-pound grass-fed lamb shoulder, trimmed and cubed into 2-inch pieces
- 1 cup fresh tomatoes, finely chopped
- 1 tablespoon fresh lemon juice
- ½ teaspoon dried basil, crushed
- ¼ cup homemade chicken broth
- 1/8 cup fresh parsley, minced
- ½ tablespoon olive oil
- 1 celery stalk, chopped
- ½ tablespoon garlic, minced

- 1 tablespoon sugar-free tomato paste
- ½ teaspoon dried oregano, crushed
- ¼ teaspoon salt and pepper
- 1 red bell pepper, quartered & seeded

How to prepare:

1. Put the olive oil and garlic in a skillet on a medium heat.
2. Sauté for about 1 minute and add onions.
3. Sauté for about 3 minutes and stir in rest of the ingredients except bell peppers and parsley.
4. Cook covered for about 30 minutes on medium-low heat.
5. Stir in the bell peppers and cook for about 5 minutes.
6. Garnish with parsley and serve hot.

Preparation time: 10 minutes

Cooking time: 40 minutes

Total time: 50 minutes

Servings: 4

Nutritional Values:

Calories 279

Total Fat 15.2 g

Saturated Fat 5.2 g

Cholesterol 99 mg

Sodium 134 mg

Total Carbs 5.4 g

Fiber 1.4 g

Sugar 3 g

Protein 29.2 g

Potassium 523 mg

Spicy Whole Chicken

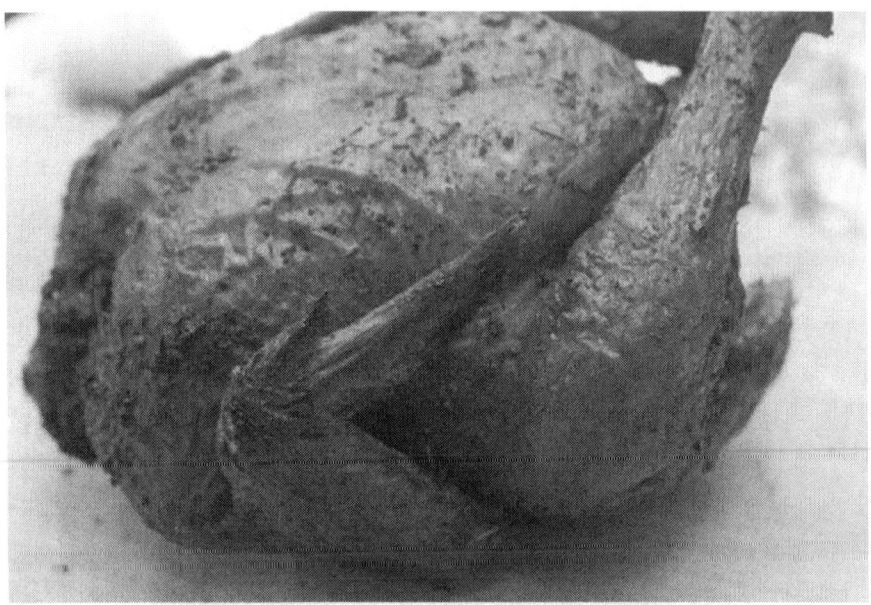

Ingredients:

- 2 teaspoons red pepper flakes, crushed
- ½ teaspoon salt and freshly ground black pepper
- 2 pounds pasture-raised whole chicken, neck and giblet removed
- 2 teaspoons ground cumin
- 1 tablespoon fresh rosemary, minced
- 2 teaspoons cayenne pepper
- 2 tablespoons olive oil

How to prepare:
1. Preheat the oven to 325 degrees F.
2. Mix together ground cumin, rosemary, cayenne pepper, red pepper flakes, salt, and black pepper.

3. Rub the chicken generously with spice mixture and sprinkle with olive oil.
4. Wrap the chicken with aluminum foil and transfer inside the oven.
5. Bake for about 40 minutes and remove from the oven.
6. Place the chicken onto a cutting board for about 10 minutes before carving.
7. Cut the chicken into desired sized pieces with a sharp knife and serve

Preparation time: 30 minutes
Cooking time: 40 minutes
Total time: 1 hour 10 minutes
Servings: 8

Nutritional Values:
Calories 249
Total Fat 18 g
Saturated Fat 5.6 g
Cholesterol 81 mg
Sodium 82 mg
Total Carbs 1 g
Fiber 0.5 g
Sugar 0.1 g
Protein 21.5 g
Potassium 32 mg

Bright Green Chicken Curry

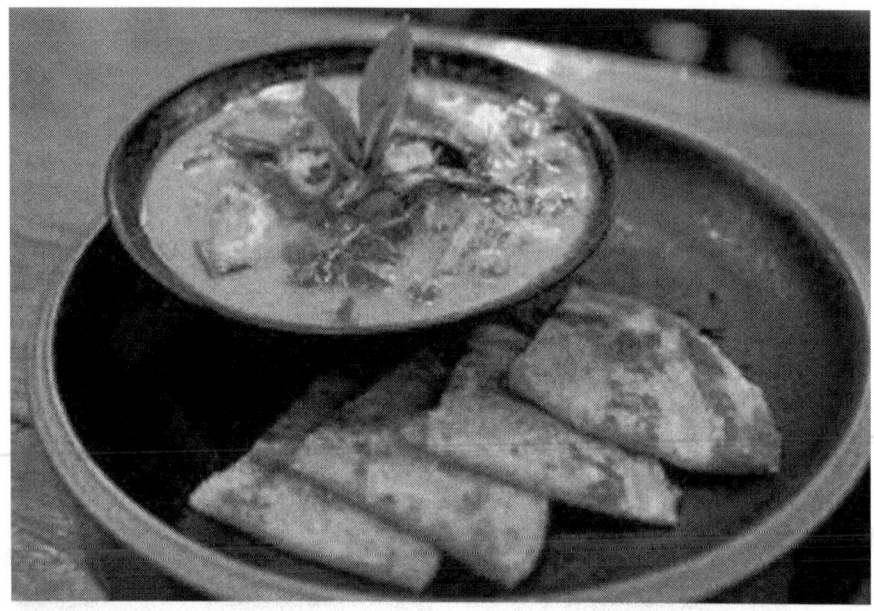

Ingredients:

- 4 pounds grass-fed boneless, skinless chicken thighs, cut into 2-inch long, thin slices
- 4 garlic cloves, crushed
- 4 tablespoons green curry paste
- 12-ounces green beans, trimmed and cut into 2-inch pieces
- 2 small yellow onion, sliced thinly
- 1 cup coconut cream
- 1 tablespoon soy sauce
- 1 tablespoon fresh lime juice
- 2 tablespoons olive oil
- 8-ounce unsweetened coconut milk

- 1 tablespoon fish sauce
- 1 cup homemade chicken broth
- ½ cup fresh cilantro, chopped
- Salt, to taste

How to prepare:
1. Rub the chicken thighs with salt and keep aside.
2. Heat the olive oil in a non-stick skillet and add garlic.
3. Sauté for about 1 minute and add onions.
4. Sauté for about 3 minutes and add coconut cream and curry paste.
5. Cook for about 4 minutes, occasionally stirring and add the coconut milk, chicken, broth and both sauces.
6. Cover the lid and cook for about 12 minutes on medium-low heat.
7. Stir in the green beans and lime juice and cook for about 3 minutes.
8. Garnish with cilantro and top with avocado slices.
9. Dish out and serve hot.

Preparation time: 15 minutes
Cooking time: 45 minutes
Total time: 1 hour
Servings: 8

Nutritional Values:

Calories 290

Total Fat 16.4 g

Saturated Fat 6.6 g

Cholesterol 108 mg

Sodium 588 mg

Total Carbs 6.6 g

Fiber 1.7 g

Sugar 1.8 g

Protein 31.5 g

Potassium 208 mg

Slow Cooker Mediterranean Stew

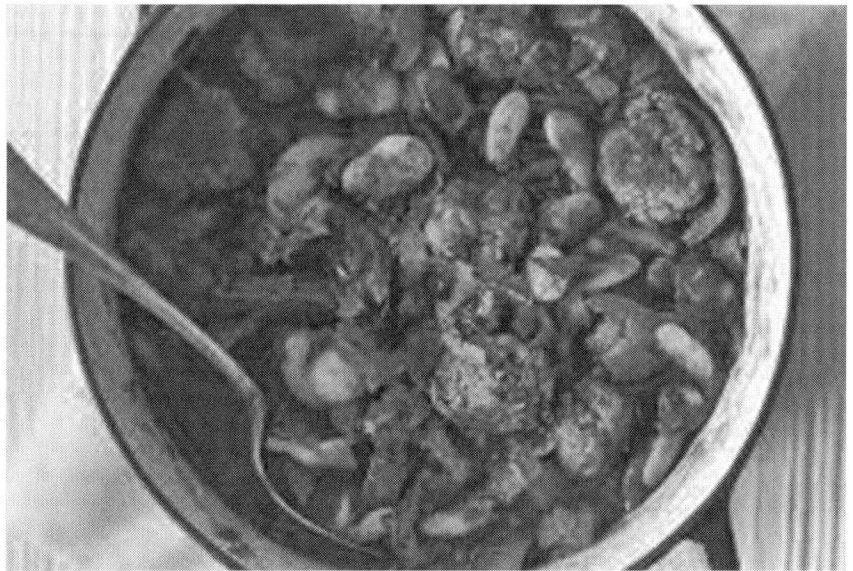

Ingredients:

- 1 cup eggplant, peeled and cubed
- ½ (8 ounce) can tomato sauce
- ½ ripe tomato, chopped
- ¼ cup vegetable broth
- ¼ teaspoon ground turmeric
- ¼ teaspoon ground cinnamon
- ½ butternut squash, peeled, seeded, and cubed
- 1 cup zucchini, cubed
- ½ (10 ounce) package frozen okra, thawed
- ½ cup onions, chopped
- ½ carrot, thinly sliced
- 1 garlic clove, chopped
- ¼ teaspoon ground cumin

- ¼ teaspoon red pepper, crushed
- ¼ teaspoon paprika

How to prepare:
1. Mix together zucchini, butternut squash, okra, onion, eggplant, tomato sauce, tomato, garlic, broth, and carrot in a slow cooker.
2. Sprinkle turmeric, cumin powder, red pepper, paprika, and cinnamon.
3. Cook covered on Low for 9 hours until the vegetables are tender.
4. Dish out and serve hot.

Preparation time: 30 minutes
Cooking time: 9 hours
Total time: 9 hours 30 minutes
Servings: 5

Nutritional Values:
Calories 40
Total Fat 0.3 g
Saturated Fat 0.1 g
Cholesterol 0 mg
Sodium 167 mg
Total Carbs 8.4 g
Fiber 2.8 g
Sugar 3.6 g
Protein 1.9 g
Potassium 356 mg

Air Fried Chicken

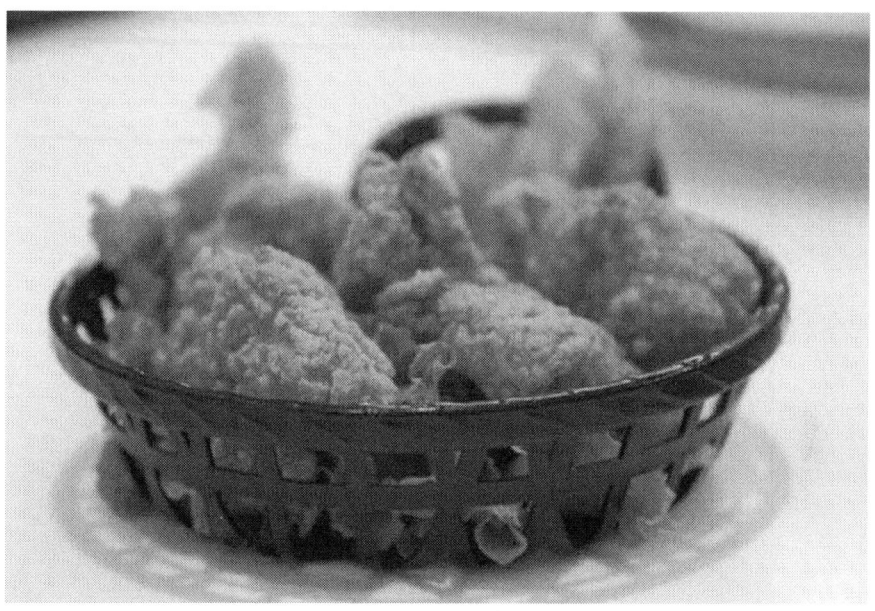

Ingredients:

- 3 tablespoons olive oil
- 1½ teaspoons turmeric powder
- 12 skinless, boneless chicken tenderloins
- ½ teaspoon salt and pepper

How to prepare:
1. Season the chicken with salt, turmeric powder, and black pepper.
2. Preheat the air fryer to 355F and coat well with olive oil.
3. Add the chicken tenderloins in the air fryer and cook for about 10 minutes.
4. Dish out and serve hot.

Preparation time: 10 minutes
Cooking time: 10 minutes
Total time: 20 minutes
Servings: 6

Nutritional Values:

Calories 342

Total Fat 14.9 g

Saturated Fat 4.4 g

Cholesterol 130 mg

Total Carbs 0.4 g

Sugar 0 g

Fiber 0.1 g

Sodium 80 mg

Potassium 14 mg

Protein 50 g

Salmon Stew

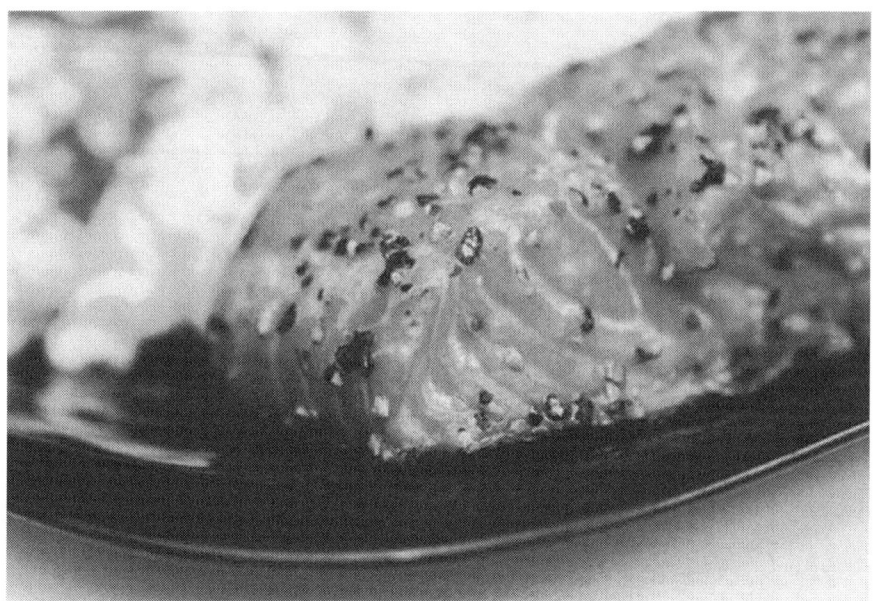

Ingredients:

- 2 medium onions, chopped
- 2 cups homemade fish broth
- 2 pounds salmon fillet, cubed
- 2 tablespoons butter
- ½ teaspoon salt and pepper

How to prepare:
1. Rub the salmon fillets with salt and black pepper.
2. Put butter and onions in a skillet on medium-high heat.
3. Sauté for about 3 minutes and add salmon.
4. Sauté 3 minutes per side and stir in fish broth.
5. Cook covered for about 6 minutes.
6. Dish out and serve hot.

Preparation time: 5 minutes
Cooking time: 11 minutes
Total time: 16 minutes
Servings: 6

Nutritional Values:
Calories 272
Total Fat 14.2 g
Saturated Fat 4.1 g
Cholesterol 82 mg
Total Carbs 4.4 g
Sugar 1.9 g
Fiber 1.1 g
Sodium 275 mg
Potassium 635 mg
Protein 32.1 g

Paprika Shrimp

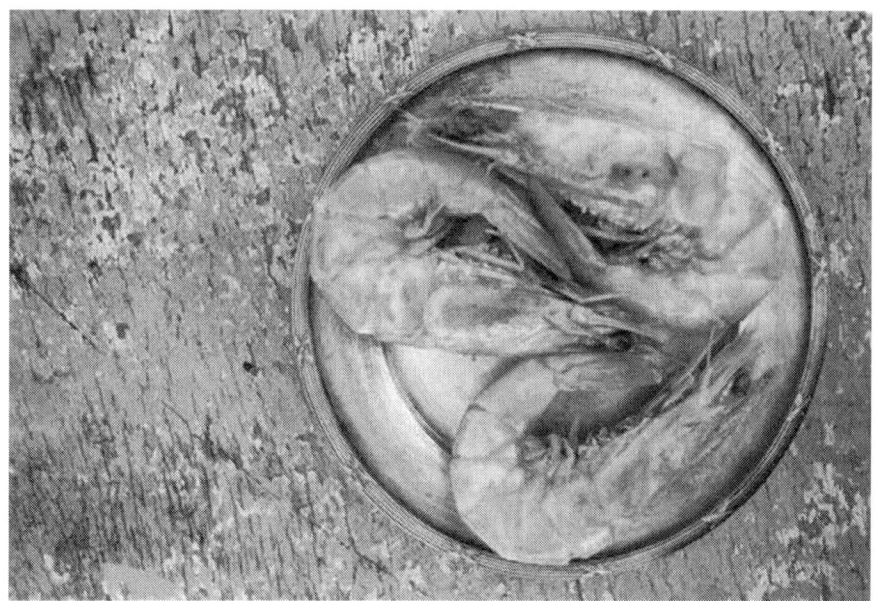

Ingredients:

- 6 tablespoons butter
- 1 teaspoon smoked paprika
- 2 pounds tiger shrimps
- Salt, to taste

How to prepare:

1. Preheat your oven to 400F.
2. In a large bowl, whisk all the listed ingredients.
3. Place the marinated shrimp in the lightly greased baking dish.

4. Transfer the baking dish in oven and bake for about 20 minutes.
5. Dish out and serve hot.

Preparation time: 5 minutes

Cooking time: 20 minutes

Total time: 25 minutes

Servings: 6

Nutritional Values:

Calories 173

Total Fat 8.3 g

Saturated Fat 1.3 g

Cholesterol 221 mg

Total Carbs 0.1 g

Sugar 0 g

Fiber 0.1 g

Sodium 332 mg

Potassium 212 mg

Protein 23.8 g

Special Butter Fish

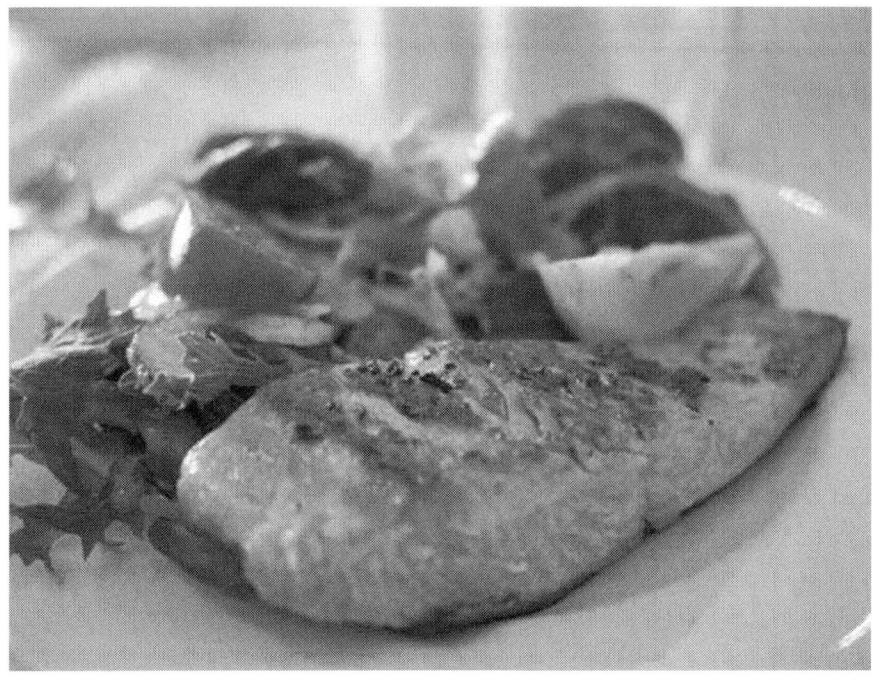

Ingredients:

- 6 green chilies, chopped
- 4 tablespoons ginger-garlic paste
- 2 pounds salmon fillets
- 1½ cups butter
- ½ teaspoon salt and freshly ground black pepper

How to prepare:
1. Season the salmon fillets with ginger-garlic paste, salt, and black pepper.
2. Place the salmon fillets in a non-stick skillet and top with the green chilies and butter.
3. Cook for 30 minutes on low heat and serve hot.

Preparation time: 10 minutes
Cooking time: 30 minutes
Total time: 40 minutes
Servings: 6

Nutritional Values:
Calories 507
Total Fat 45.9 g
Saturated Fat 22.9 g
Cholesterol 142 mg
Total Carbs 2.4 g
Sugar 0.2 g
Fiber 0.1 g
Sodium 296 mg
Potassium 453 mg
Protein 22.8 g

DINNER RECIPES

Harvested Chicken Stew

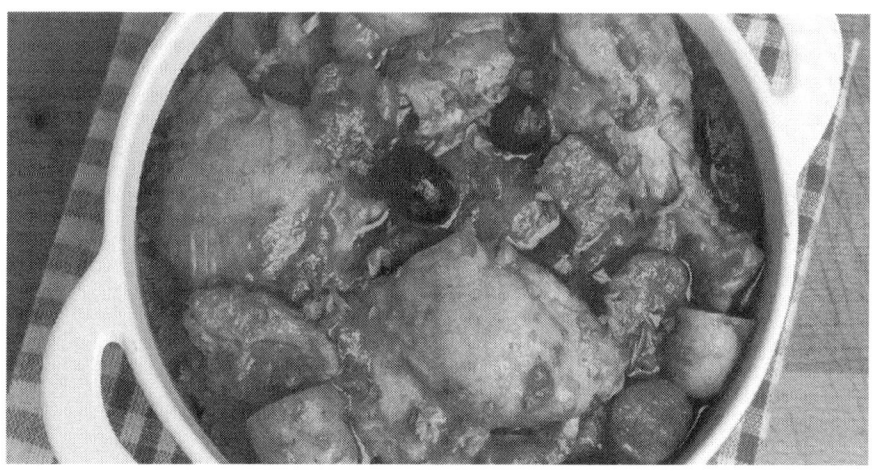

Ingredients:

- 1 cup boneless chicken breast meat, cubed and cooked
- 1 cup tomatoes, whole peeled
- ¼ cup corns
- ½ cup zucchini, sliced
- 1 cup onions, chopped
- ½ cup celery, chopped
- ¾ cup carrots, sliced
- 2½ cups chicken broth
- ¼ cup peas

How to prepare:
1. Mix together chicken, celery, onions, tomatoes, peas, corn, zucchini, broth, and carrots in a large soup pot.
2. Mix gently and allow it to simmer on medium low heat for 30 minutes.
3. Dish out and serve hot.

Preparation time: 15 minutes
Cooking time: 30 minutes
Total time: 45 minutes
Servings: 5

Nutritional Values:
Calories 143
Total Fat 3.4 g
Saturated Fat 0.9 g
Cholesterol 13 mg
Sodium 1642 mg
Total Carbs 10.3 g
Fiber 2.2 g
Sugar 4.1 g
Protein 16.9 g
Potassium 699 mg

Shrimp Curry

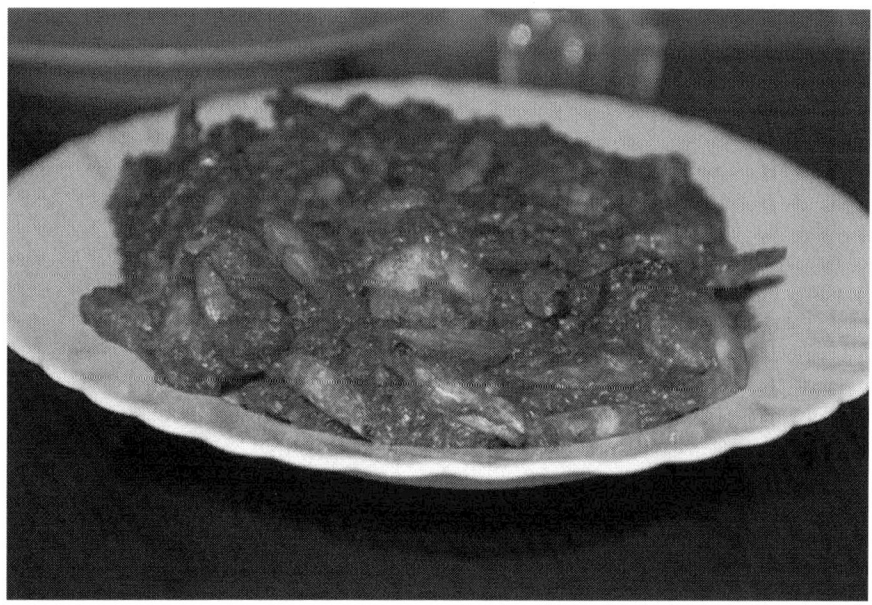

Ingredients:

- ½ teaspoon ground turmeric
- ½ tablespoon olive oil
- ¾ teaspoon red chili powder
- 1 pound medium shrimp, peeled and deveined
- ½ tablespoon fresh lemon juice
- ½ medium onion, chopped
- Pinch of salt
- ¼ cup water
- ¼ teaspoon ground cumin
- 1 medium tomato, chopped
- 1/8 cup fresh cilantro, chopped

How to prepare:
1. Sauté garlic, onions, carrot, bell pepper, and celery in heated oil for about 3 minutes and add turmeric, red chili powder, salt, and cumin.
2. Cook 1 more minute and add tomatoes and water.
3. Cook for about 3 minutes and stir in the shrimp.
4. Cook covered for about 5 minutes on medium-high heat.
5. Dish out and serve hot.

Preparation time: 10 minutes
Cooking time: 12 minutes
Total time: 22 minutes
Servings: 3

Nutritional Values:

Calories 189

Total Fat 4.7 g

Saturated Fat 0.4 g

Cholesterol 297 mg

Sodium 397 mg

Total Carbs 5 g

Fiber 1.8 g

Sugar 2.1 g

Protein 33.3 g

Potassium 189 mg

Mexican Beef Brisket

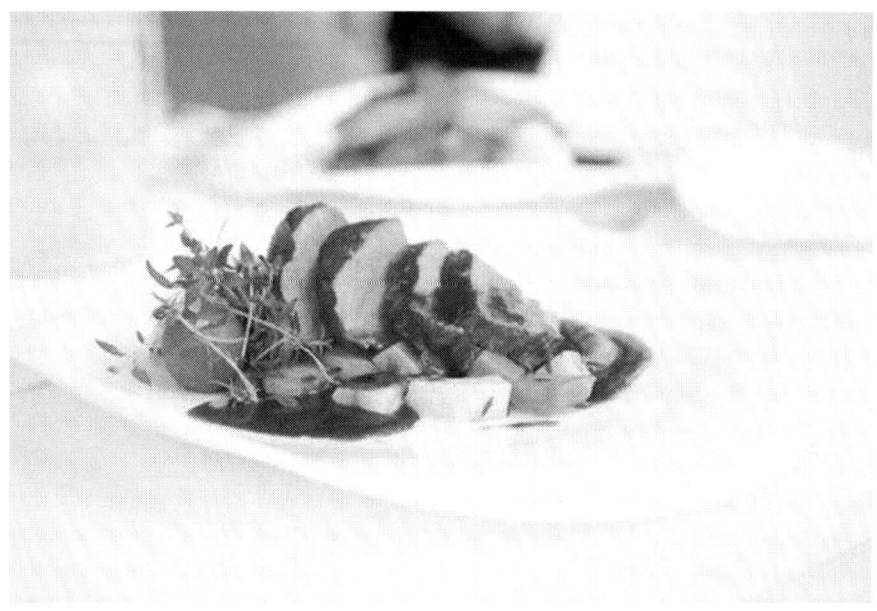

Ingredients:

- 1 tablespoon chili powder
- 3 pounds grass-fed beef boneless brisket, trimmed and cut into 1½-inch cubes
- 1 tablespoon olive oil
- 1 cup homemade beef broth
- 1 tablespoon sugar-free tomato paste
- 1 onion, sliced thinly
- 1 teaspoon salt and freshly pepper
- ½ cup roasted tomato salsa
- 6 garlic cloves, peeled and smashed

How to prepare:
1. Mix together beef, chili powder, salt, and black pepper together in a large bowl.
2. Put the olive oil and onions in a pressure cooker.
3. Sauté for 2 minutes and add tomato paste and garlic.
4. Sauté for about 1 minute and add beef, salsa, and broth.
5. Lock the lid and cook for 25 minutes at high pressure.
6. Naturally release the pressure and dish out.

Preparation time: 5 minutes
Cooking time: 28 minutes
Total time: 33 minutes
Servings: 10

Nutritional Values:
Calories 259
Total Fat 18.6 g
Saturated Fat 7.5 g
Cholesterol 85 mg
Sodium 1359 mg
Total Carbs 3.2 g
Fiber 0.6 g
Sugar 0.7 g
Protein 18.9 g
Potassium 264 mg

Citrus Glazed Salmon

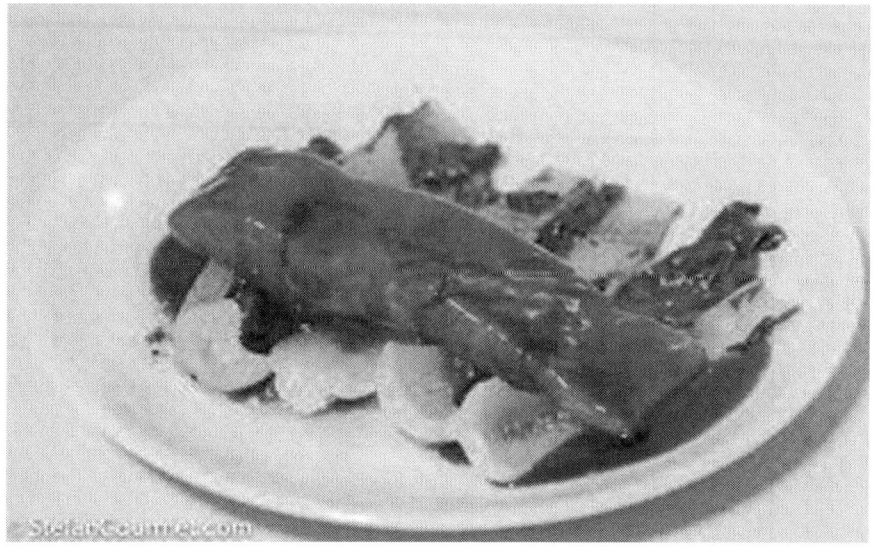

Ingredients:

- 1 cup white wine
- Freshly ground black pepper, to taste
- 2 tablespoons fresh orange juice
- 1 teaspoon fresh ginger, minced
- 1 tablespoon olive oil
- 4 (2-ounce) salmon fillets
- 2 teaspoons fresh orange zest, grated finely

How to prepare:

1. In a medium-sized glass bowl, whisk together all the ingredients excluding the salmon fillets.
2. Marinate the salmon in this mixture for about 1 hour.
3. Put the marinated salmon fillets in a non-stick pan.

4. Cook for about 15 minutes on both sides, occasionally flipping.
5. Top with cooking sauce and serve.

Preparation time: 30 minutes
Cooking time: 15 minutes
Total time: 45 minutes
Servings: 4

Nutritional Values:

Calories 160
Total Fat 7.1 g
Saturated Fat 1 g
Cholesterol 25 mg
Sodium 28 mg
Total Carbs 3 g
Fiber 0.2 g
Sugar 1.1 g
Protein 11.2 g
Potassium 48 mg

Beef Bulgogi

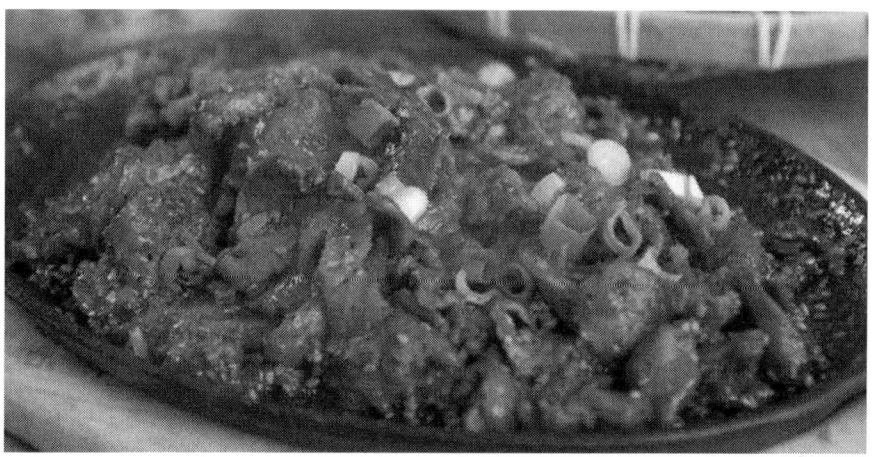

Ingredients:

- ½ cup green onion, chopped
- 2 teaspoons Splenda
- 4 tablespoons olive oil
- 10 tablespoons soy sauce
- 2 pounds flank steak, thinly sliced
- 4 tablespoons garlic, minced
- 1 teaspoon freshly ground black pepper

How to prepare:
1. Mix together beef, green onion, soy sauce, garlic, olive oil, sugar, and black pepper in a bowl and keep aside for 1 hour.
2. Preheat a grill on high heat and grease the grate with oil lightly.
3. Grill the beef 3 minutes on each side and serve.

Preparation time: 15 minutes
Cooking time: 6 minutes
Total time: 21 minutes
Servings: 8

Nutritional Values:
Calories 330
Total Fat 18.5 g
Saturated Fat 5.2 g
Cholesterol 62 mg
Sodium 1193 mg
Total Carbs 5.6 g
Fiber 1 g
Sugar 1.5 g
Protein 34 g
Potassium 485 mg

Delicious Lobster

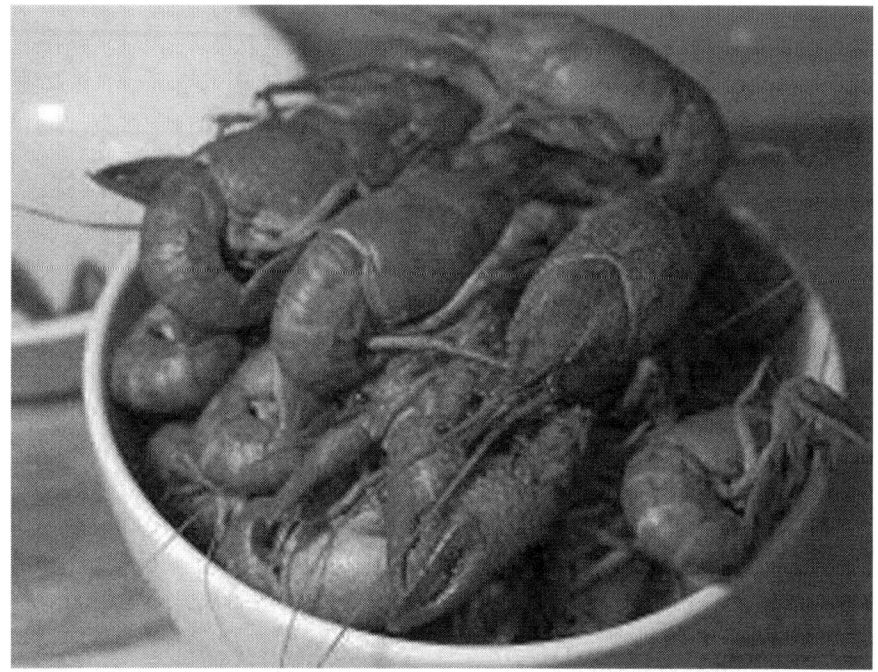

Ingredients:

- ½ teaspoon old bay seasoning
- ¼ cup mayonnaise
- 1 tablespoon fresh lemon juice, divided
- ¾ cup water
- 1 tablespoon unsalted butter, melted
- 1 pound fresh lobster tails
- ½ scallion, chopped

How to prepare:
1. Arrange the steamer basket in the pressure cooker and add water and half of old bay seasoning.

2. Place lobster tails on the steamer basket, meat side up.
3. Drizzle lobster tails with half of lemon juice and cook on high pressure for about 3 minutes.
4. Quickly release the pressure and remove the meat.
5. Chop it up into large chunks and add in a large bowl along with scallions, mayonnaise, butter, leftover bay seasoning, and remaining lemon juice.

Preparation time: 20 minutes
Cooking time: 3 minutes
Total time: 23 minutes
Servings: 3

Nutritional Values:
Calories 247
Total Fat 11.7 g
Saturated Fat 3.7 g
Cholesterol 236 mg
Sodium 1016 mg
Total Carbs 5 g
Fiber 0.1 g
Sugar 1.4 g
Protein 29 g
Potassium 519 mg

Cheesy Cauliflower

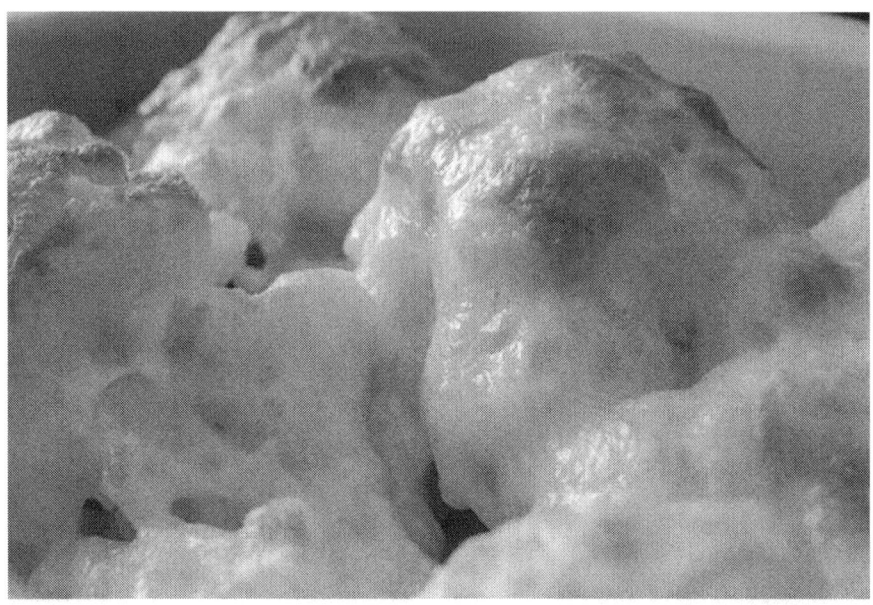

Ingredients:

- ½ cup butter, cut into small pieces
- 2 tablespoons prepared mustard
- 2 cauliflower heads
- 2 teaspoons mayonnaise
- 1 cup parmesan cheese, grated

How to prepare:

1. Preheat the oven to 390F and grease a small baking dish.
2. Mix together mustard and mayonnaise in a bowl.
3. Coat the cauliflower head with the mustard mixture and arrange in a baking dish.

4. Top evenly with butter and cheese.
5. Sprinkle with cheese evenly and bake for about 25 minutes.
6. Dish out and serve hot.

Preparation time: 10 minutes
Cooking time: 20 minutes
Total time: 30 minutes
Servings: 6

Nutritional Values:
Calories 183
Total Fat 17.2 g
Saturated Fat 10.5 g
Cholesterol 44 mg
Total Carbs 5.5 g
Sugar 2.3 g
Fiber 2.4 g
Sodium 250 mg
Potassium 280 mg
Protein 3.7 g

Jamaican Jerk Pork Roast

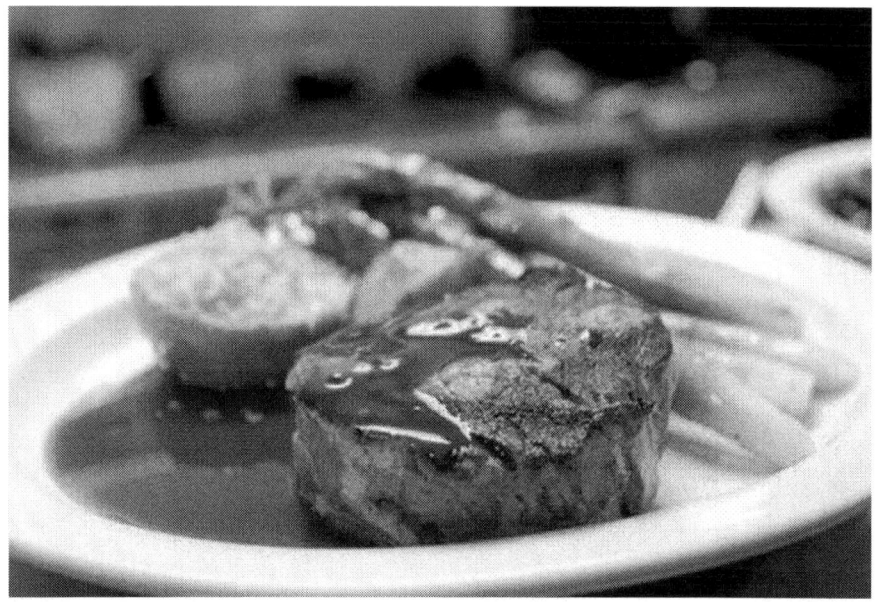

Ingredients:

- 1 tablespoon butter
- ¼ cup Jamaican jerk spice blend
- 1 pound pork shoulder
- ¼ cup beef broth

How to prepare:
1. Rub the pork with Jamaican jerk spice blend.
2. Heat the butter in the pot and add seasoned pork.
3. Cook for about 5 minutes and add beef broth.
4. Cook covered for about 20 minutes on low heat.
5. Dish out and serve hot.

Preparation time: 10 minutes
Cooking time: 25 minutes
Total time: 35 minutes
Servings: 3

Nutritional Values:
Calories 477
Total Fat 36.2 g
Saturated Fat 14.3 g
Cholesterol 146 mg
Total Carbs 0 g
Sugar 0 g
Fiber 0 g
Sodium 162 mg
Potassium 507 mg
Protein 35.4 g

Pork Carnitas

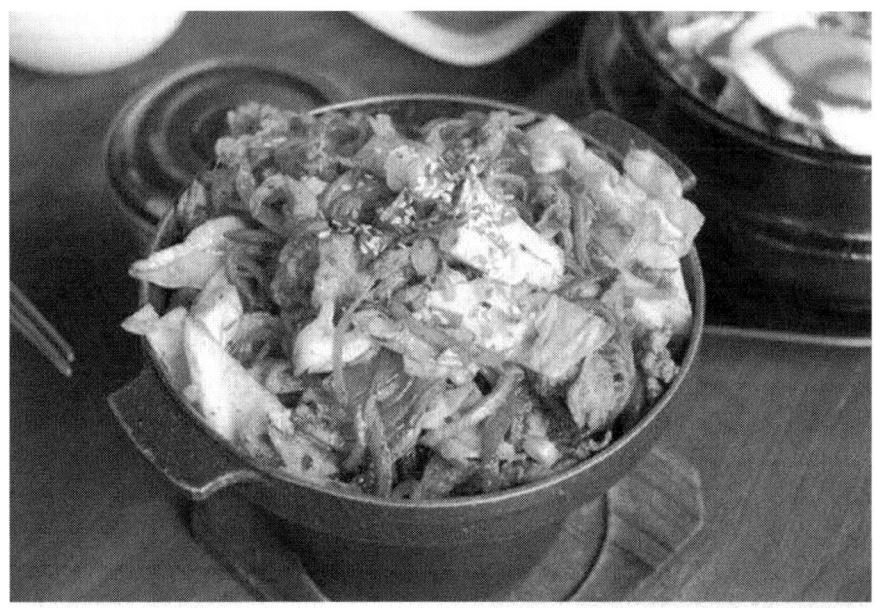

Ingredients:

- 2 oranges, juiced
- 2 tablespoons butter
- 2 pounds pork shoulder, bone-in
- 1 teaspoon garlic powder
- ½ teaspoon salt and pepper

How to prepare:

1. Rub the pork with garlic powder, salt, and black pepper.
2. Put butter and seasoned pork in the pressure cooker.
3. Sauté for about 3 minutes and stir in orange juice.

4. Secure the lid and cook for about 8 minutes at high pressure.

5. Naturally release the pressure and dish out.

Preparation time: 10 minutes

Cooking time: 12 minutes

Total time: 22 minutes

Servings: 6

Nutritional Values:

Calories 506

Total Fat 36.3 g

Saturated Fat 14.3 g

Cholesterol 146 mg

Total carbs 7.6 g

Sugar 5.8 g

Fiber 1.5 g

Sodium 130 mg

Potassium 615 mg

Protein 35.9 g

SOUP RECIPES

Omega-3 Rich Salmon Soup

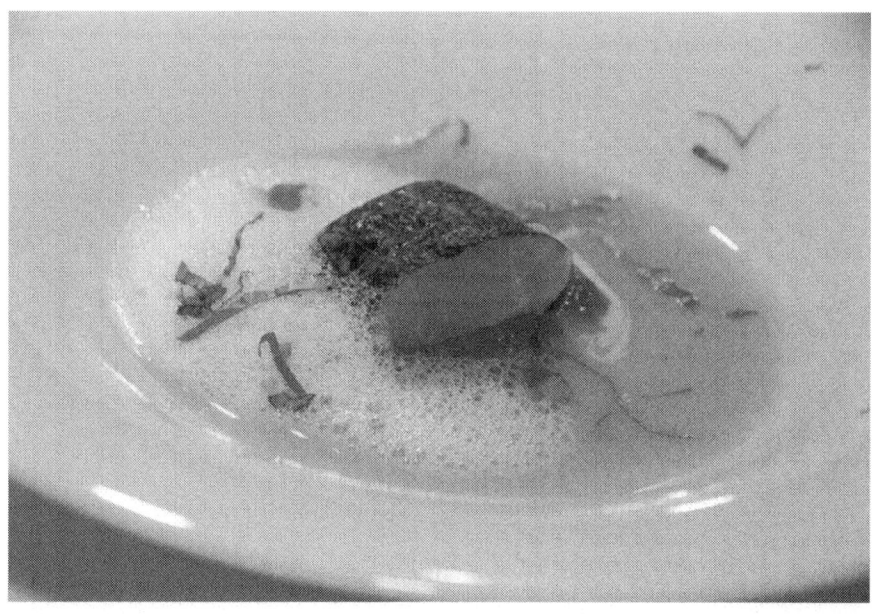

Ingredients:

- 1 cup celery, chopped
- 2 cups carrots, peeled and chopped
- 2 cups cauliflowers, chopped
- ½ cup fresh parsley, chopped
- 2 tablespoons coconut oil
- 4 cups homemade chicken broth
- 2 pounds salmon fillets
- 1 cup yellow onions, chopped
- 1 teaspoon salt and pepper

How to prepare:
1. Put the coconut oil and salmon fillets in a wok.
2. Cook 3 minutes per side and add onions, carrots, and cauliflowers.
3. Cook for 2 more minutes and add celery stalk, chicken broth, salt, and black pepper.
4. Cover the lid and cook for about 18 minutes on medium-low heat.
5. Dish out the salmon fillets and cut into small pieces.
6. Return the salmon chunks to the wok and allow it to simmer for about 5 minutes.
7. Garnish with fresh parsley and dish out to serve hot.

Preparation time: 15 minutes
Cooking time: 30 minutes
Total time: 45 minutes
Servings: 8

Nutritional Values:
Calories 225
Total Fat 11.2 g
Saturated Fat 4.1 g
Cholesterol 50 mg
Sodium 471 mg
Total Carbs 6.5 g
Fiber 1.9 g
Sugar 3.1 g
Protein 25.5 g
Potassium 417 mg

Cheesy Broccoli Soup

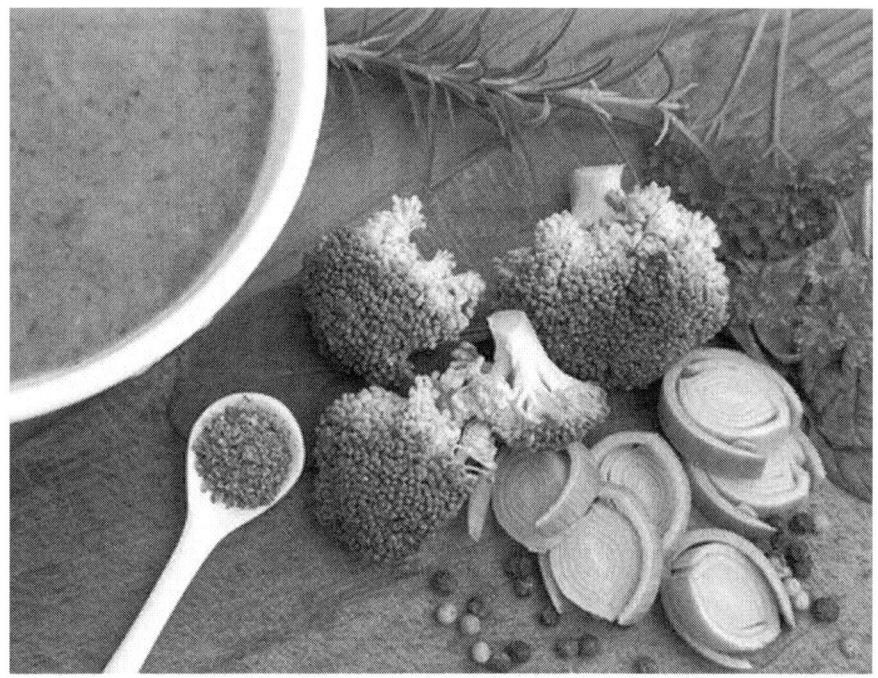

Ingredients:

- 2 cups chicken broth
- 1 cup heavy whipping cream
- 2 cups broccoli
- 2 cups cheddar cheese
- Salt, to taste

How to prepare:

1. Stir in the chicken broth, broccoli, cheddar cheese, salt, and heavy whipping cream in the slow cooker.
2. Set on low and simmer for about 4 hours.
3. Dish out and serve simmering hot.

Preparation time: 10 minutes
Cooking time: 4 hours
Total time: 4 hours 10 minutes
Servings: 6

Nutritional Values:
Calories 244
Total Fat 20.4 g
Saturated Fat 67 g
Cholesterol 130 mg
Total Carbs 3.4 g
Sugar 1 g
Fiber 0.8 g
Sodium 506 mg
Potassium 217 mg
Protein 12.3 g

Egg Soup

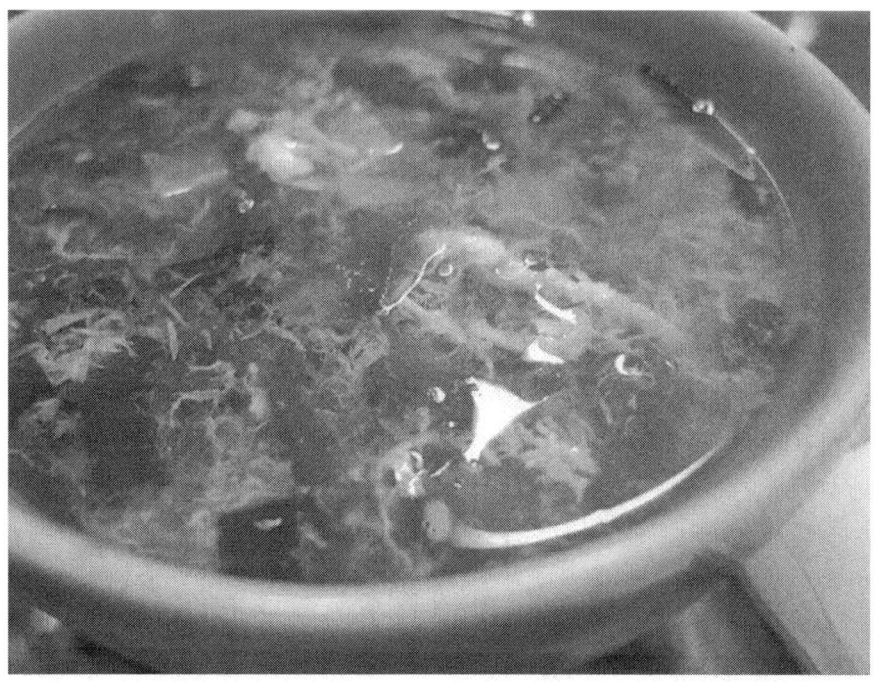

Ingredients:

- 2 eggs
- 6 cups chicken broth, divided
- 1 tablespoon arrowroot powder
- 1 tablespoon garlic, minced
- ½ cup fresh lemon juice
- 1 tablespoon olive oil
- ¼ teaspoon salt and white pepper

How to prepare:
1. Mix together lemon juice, arrowroot powder, eggs, salt, white pepper, and 2 cups broth in a bowl.

2. Put oil and garlic in a large soup pan over medium-high heat.
3. Sauté for about 2 minutes and add rest of the broth.
4. Boil and simmer on low for about 6 minutes and add egg mixture slowly in the pan, continuously stirring.
5. Cook 5 minutes more and serve hot in soup bowls.

Preparation time: 15 minutes
Cooking time: 13 minutes
Total time: 28 minutes
Servings: 6

Nutritional Values:
Calories 92
Total Fat 5.3 g
Saturated Fat 1.3 g
Cholesterol 55 mg
Sodium 788 mg
Total Carbs 3.2 g
Fiber 0.1 g
Sugar 1.3 g
Protein 7 g
Potassium 257 mg

Asparagus Soup

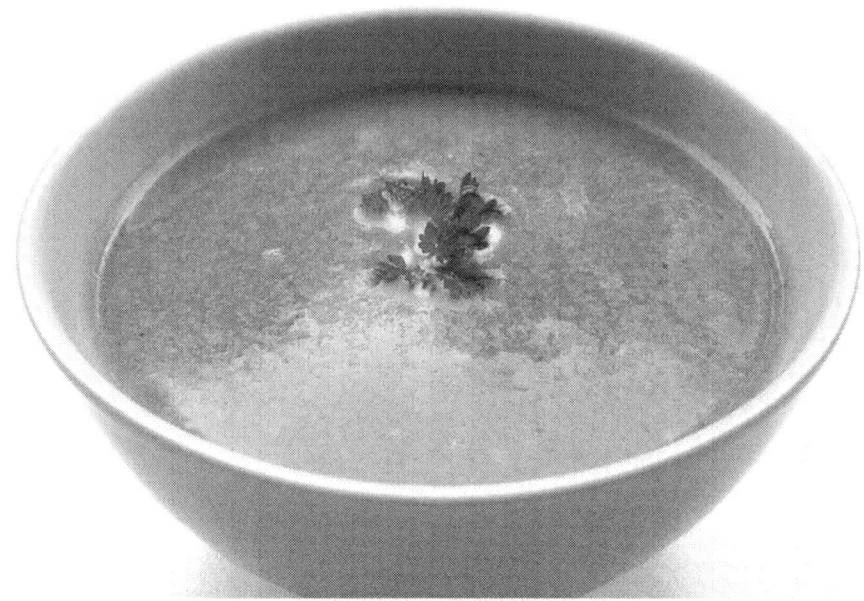

Ingredients:

- 2 scallions, chopped
- 2 tablespoons fresh lemon juice
- 1 tablespoon olive oil
- 1 pound asparagus, trimmed and chopped
- 4 cups vegetable broth
- ¼ teaspoon salt and pepper

How to prepare:
1. Heat oil and scallions in a large pan over medium heat.
2. Sauté for about 5 minutes and add asparagus and broth.
3. Boil and lower the flame.

4. Cook 30 minutes. Let it cool slightly off the stove and add soup in batches in an immersion blender.
5. Pulse until smooth and return the soup into the pan.
6. Simmer for about 5 minutes and stir in the lemon juice, salt, and black pepper.
7. Remove from heat and serve hot.

Preparation time: 15 minutes
Cooking time: 10 minutes
Total time: 25 minutes
Servings: 4

Nutritional Values:
Calories 95
Total Fat 5.1 g
Saturated Fat 1 g
Cholesterol 0 mg
Sodium 768 mg
Total Carbs 6 g
Fiber 2.6 g
Sugar 3.2 g
Protein 7.5 g
Potassium 466 mg

Chicken & Lime Soup

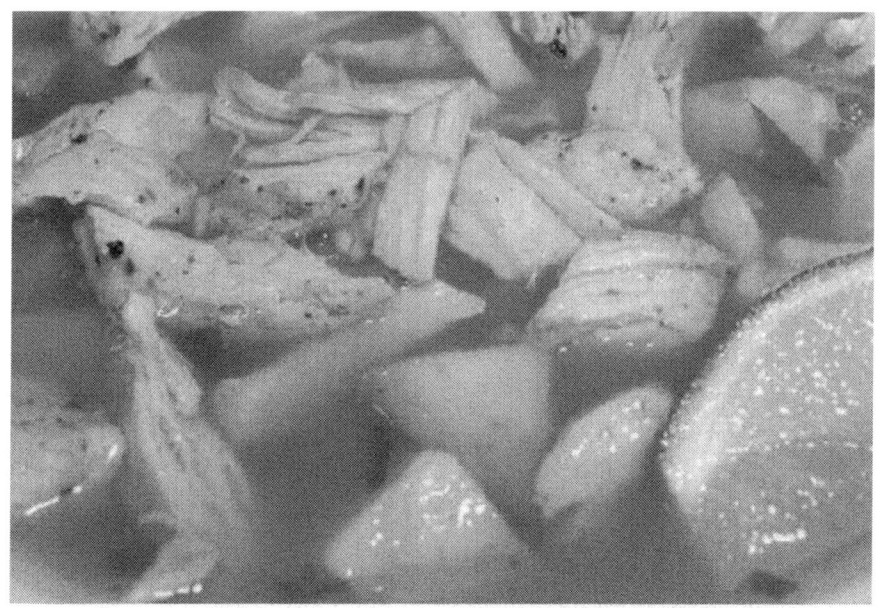

Ingredients:

- 2 small onions, chopped
- 2 medium tomatoes, chopped
- ½ cup fresh lime juice
- 1 teaspoon ground cumin
- 1 teaspoon red chili powder
- 4 cups boneless chicken, cubed
- 8 garlic cloves, minced
- 12-ounce mushrooms, chopped
- 8 cups chicken broth
- 1 teaspoon oregano
- ¼ teaspoon salt and pepper

How to prepare:
1. In a slow cooker, combine all ingredients and mix.
2. Set the slow cooker over low and cook covered for about 8 hours.
3. Transfer the chicken into a bowl and shred it with the help of 2 forks.
4. Transfer the chicken into soup and stir well to serve immediately.

Preparation time: 20 minutes
Cooking time: 8 hours
Total time: 8 hours 20 minutes
Servings: 10

Nutritional Values:
Calories 161
Total Fat 5.5 g
Saturated Fat 1.5 g
Cholesterol 50 mg
Sodium 666 mg
Total Carbs 5.4 g
Fiber 1.2 g
Sugar 2.5 g
Protein 21.8 g
Potassium 512 mg

Beef & Veggies Soup

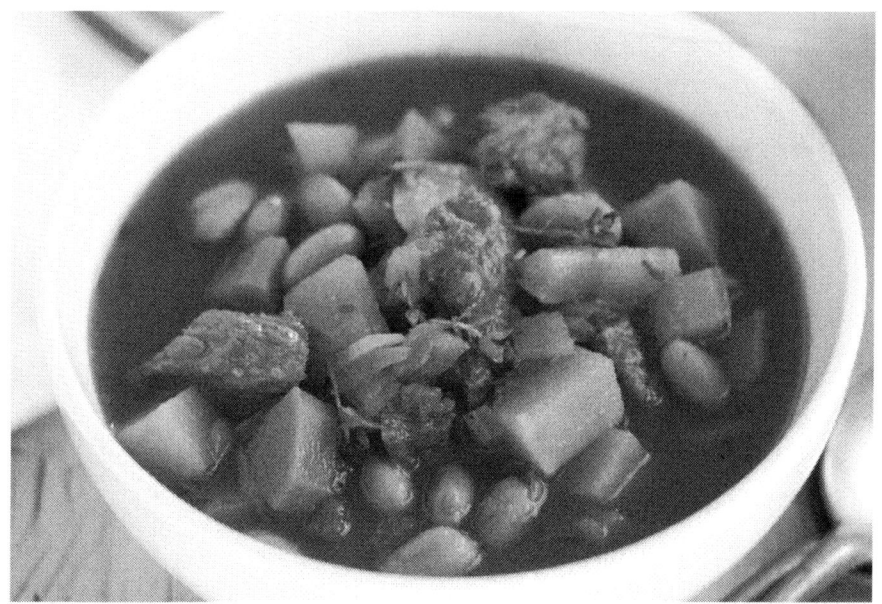

Ingredients:

- 8 cups water
- 4 scallions, chopped (reserved green part)
- 10 garlic cloves, minced
- 1 teaspoon red pepper flakes, crushed
- 2 lemons, sliced
- 8 cups chicken broth
- 6 cups broccoli, chopped
- 16-ounce mushrooms, sliced
- 2 (1-inch) pieces fresh ginger, minced
- 2 pounds cooked beef, sliced thinly
- 6 tablespoons coconut aminos

How to prepare:
1. Put broth in a pan and bring to a boil.
2. Add broccoli and cook for about 2 minutes.
3. Stir in scallions, mushrooms, garlic and ginger and simmer for about 8 minutes.
4. Add beef, red pepper flakes and coconut aminos and stir well.
5. Simmer on low for about 5 minutes.
6. Garnish with the lemon slices and reserved green part of scallion and serve hot.

Preparation time: 20 minutes
Cooking time: 15 minutes
Total time: 35 minutes
Servings: 8

Nutritional Values:
Calories 310
Total Fat 9 g
Saturated Fat 3.1 g
Cholesterol 101 mg
Sodium 886 mg
Total Carbs 13.1 g
Fiber 3.2 g
Sugar 3.4 g
Protein 43.6 g
Potassium 1128 mg

Salmon Soup

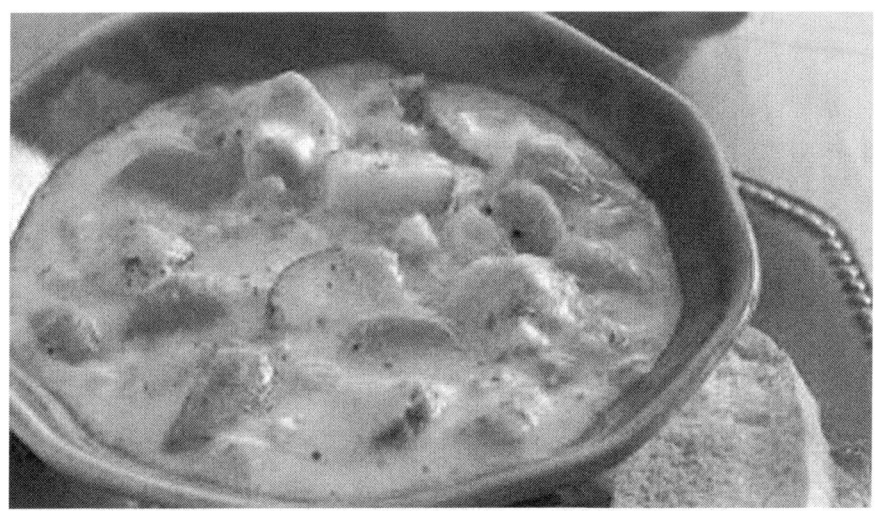

Ingredients:

- 2 onions, chopped
- 2 pounds boneless salmon, cubed
- 4 tablespoons of fresh cilantro, chopped
- 2 tablespoons fresh lime juice
- 2 tablespoons olive oil
- 2 garlic cloves, minced
- 8 cups chicken broth
- 2 tablespoons tamari
- Freshly ground black pepper, to taste

How to prepare:

1. Sauté onions in a Dutch oven for about 5 minutes and add garlic and lime leaves.
2. Sauté for about 1 minute and add broth.

3. Boil and simmer on low.
4. Simmer for about 15 minutes and add tamari and salmon.
5. Cook for about 4 minutes and stir in black pepper, lime juice, and cilantro.
6. Dish out and serve hot.

Preparation time: 20 minutes
Cooking time: 25 minutes
Total time: 45 minutes
Servings: 10

Nutritional Values:
Calories 234
Total Fat 11.3 g
Saturated Fat 1.9 g
Cholesterol 64 mg
Sodium 864 mg
Total Carbs 3.9 g
Fiber 0.6 g
Sugar 1.7 g
Protein 27.7 g
Potassium 789 mg

Ground Beef Soup

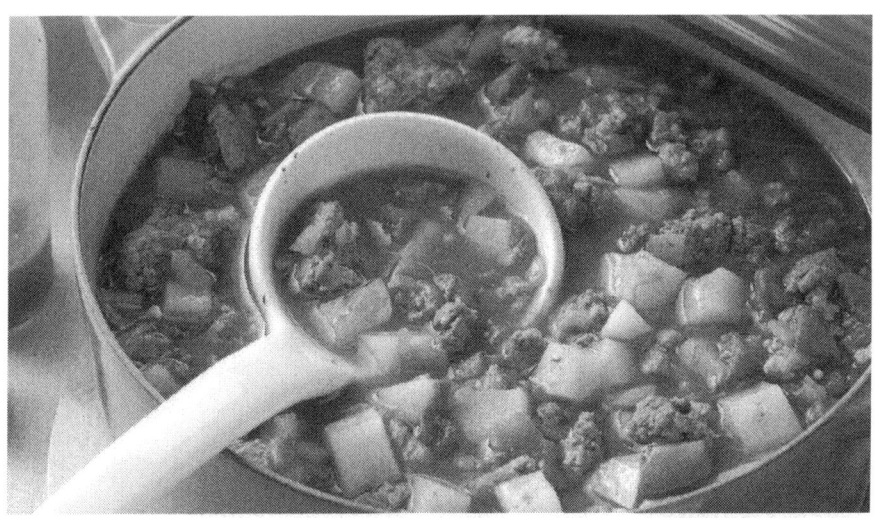

Ingredients:

- ¼ pound fresh mushrooms, sliced
- ½ teaspoon fresh ginger, minced
- 1 tablespoon soy sauce
- 2 cups chicken broth
- ½ pound lean ground beef
- ½ small onion, chopped
- 1 garlic clove, minced
- ½ pound head Bok Choy, stalks and leaves separated and chopped
- Ground black pepper, to taste

How to prepare:
1. Heat a large non-stick soup pan over medium-high heat and add beef.

2. Cook for about 5 minutes and add onion, mushrooms, and garlic.
3. Cook for about 5 minutes and add Bok Choy stalks.
4. Cook for about 5 minutes and add soy sauce and broth.
5. Bring to a boil and reduce the heat to low.
6. Simmer, covered for about 10 minutes and stir in Bok Choy leaves.
7. Simmer for about 5 minutes and stir in black pepper.

Preparation time: 20 minutes
Cooking time: 30 minutes
Total time: 50 minutes
Servings: 3

Nutritional Values:

Calories 193

Total Fat 6 g

Saturated Fat 2.1 g

Cholesterol 68 mg

Sodium 911 mg

Total Carbs 5.5 g

Fiber 1.5 g

Sugar 2.1 g

Protein 29 g

Potassium 790 mg

Shrimp Soup

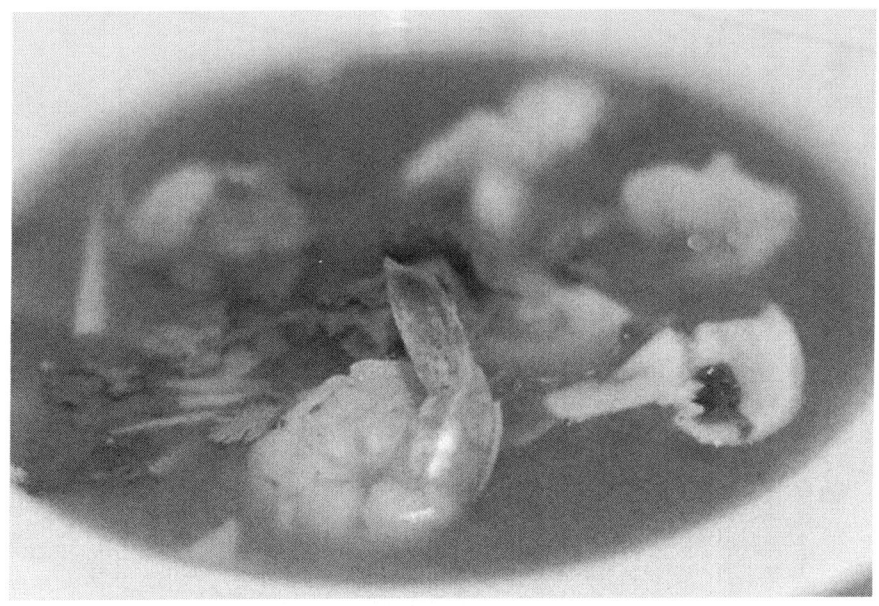

Ingredients:

- 1 fresh red chile, sliced
- ½ tablespoon fresh ginger, sliced
- 1 tablespoon fish sauce
- ¼ cup fresh cilantro, chopped
- 1 scallion, sliced
- 4 cups chicken broth
- 2 kaffir lime leaves
- 6-ounce canned straw mushrooms, halved
- ½ pound large shrimp, peeled and deveined
- 1/8 cup fresh lime juice

How to prepare:
1. Put broth in a large pan and bring to a boil over medium-high heat.
2. Stir in ginger, red chilies, lemongrass stalks, and lime leaves and reduce the heat to medium-low.
3. Simmer, covered for about 15 minutes and add mushrooms and fish sauce.
4. Simmer, uncovered for about 7 minutes and add shrimps.
5. Cook for about 8 minutes and stir in remaining ingredients.
6. Remove from heat and serve immediately.

Preparation time: 20 minutes
Cooking time: 25 minutes
Total time: 45 minutes
Servings: 3

Nutritional Values:
Calories 151
Total Fat 2.3 g
Saturated Fat 0.6 g
Cholesterol 108 mg
Sodium 1808 mg
Total Carbs 9.6 g
Fiber 1.7 g
Sugar 2 g
Protein 23.7 g
Potassium 372 mg

DESSERTS RECIPES

Berries and Cream

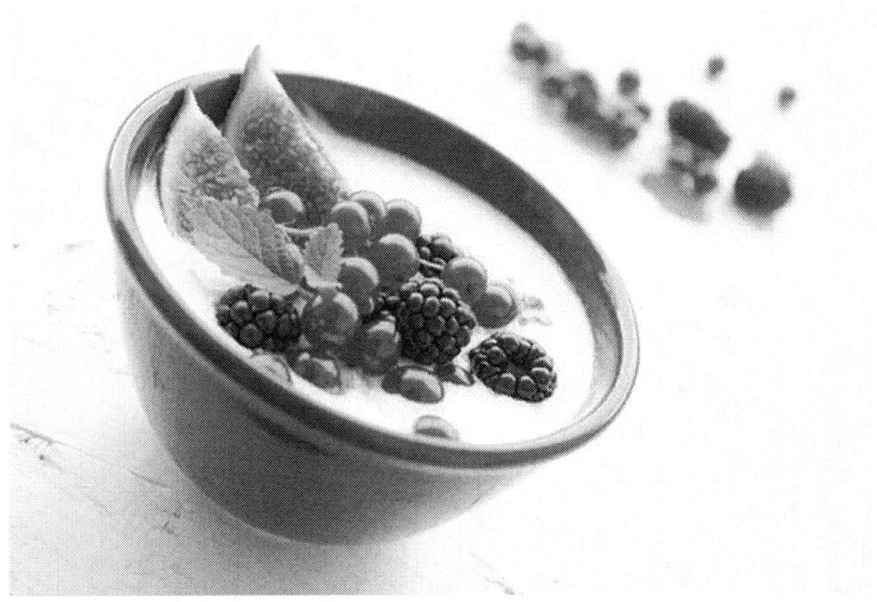

Ingredients:

- ½ cup fresh blueberries
- ½ tablespoon nonfat evaporated milk
- ¾ tablespoon Marsala wine
- ¾ cup fresh strawberries, sliced
- ½ cup ricotta cheese, part-skim
- 1 scoop stevia
- ¼ cup cream
- ¾ tablespoon hazelnuts, toasted and chopped

How to prepare:
1. Layer the strawberries and blueberries in serving bowls.
2. Whip together the cream, ricotta cheese, milk, stevia, and wine with an electric beater.
3. Place a portion of the cream over the fruits and layer with toasted hazelnuts.
4. Chill before serving.

Preparation time: 5 minutes
Cooking time: 10 minutes
Total time: 15 minutes
Servings: 3

Nutritional Values:
Calories 108
Total Fat 5.3 g
Saturated Fat 2.8 g
Cholesterol 17 mg
Sodium 62 mg
Total Carbs 9.6 g
Fiber 1.4 g
Sugar 5.1 g
Protein 5.7 g
Potassium 154 mg

Fresh Strawberry Granita

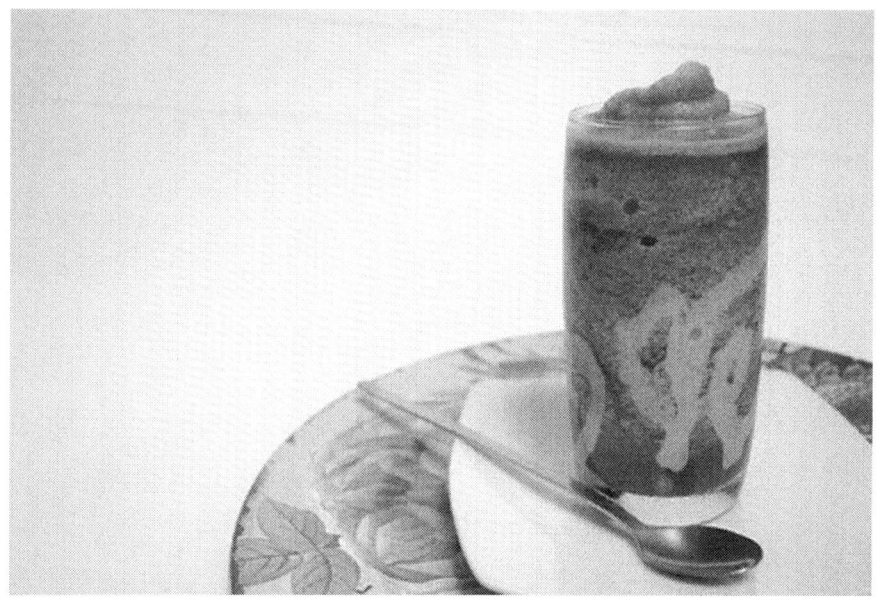

Ingredients:

- 1 scoop stevia
- ¼ teaspoon lemon juice
- ½ pinch salt
- ½ pound ripe strawberries, hulled and halved
- ½ cup water
- 1/8 teaspoon balsamic vinegar

How to prepare:
1. Rinse strawberries with cold water and drain thoroughly.
2. Transfer the berries into a blender and add balsamic vinegar, stevia, water, salt, and lemon juice.
3. Pulse until the mixture is smooth and pour into a large baking dish.

4. Transfer the dish in the freezer uncovered for about 45 minutes until the mixture begins to freeze around the edges.
5. Stir the crystals lightly from the edge into the center of the granita mixture with a fork.
6. Mix thoroughly and chill until granita is nearly frozen for about 40 more minutes.
7. Mix with a fork lightly scraping the crystals loose as before.
8. Repeat freezing and stirring with the fork 3 to 4 times until the crystals are separate.
9. Divide the granita into small serving bowls to serve.

Preparation time: 10 minutes
Cooking time: 0 minutes
Total time: 10 minutes
Servings: 4

Nutritional Values:
Calories 21
Total Fat 0.2 g
Saturated Fat 0 g
Cholesterol 0 mg
Sodium 21 mg
Total Carbs 4.9 g
Fiber 1.1 g
Sugar 3.3 g
Protein 0.4 g
Potassium 88 mg

Limeabalemon Glaciate

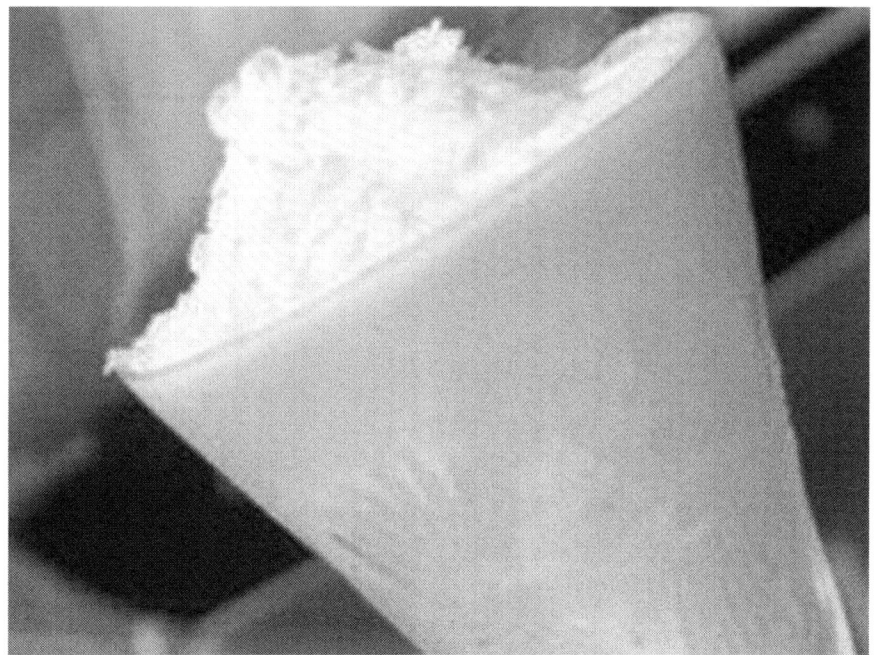

Ingredients:

- 1 ripe banana
- 1 lemon, juiced
- 3 cups crushed ice
- 1 lime, juiced
- 3 pitted cherries, as garnish

How to prepare:
1. Blend the banana and ice in a blender until completely smooth.
2. Add lemon juice and lime juice to keep the ice from freezing to the side of the blender.
3. Garnish with a cherry in serving glasses and serve.

Preparation time: 15 minutes
Cooking time: 30 minutes
Total time: 45 minutes
Servings: 3

Nutritional Values:
Calories 48
Total Fat 0.2 g
Saturated Fat 0 g
Cholesterol 0 mg
Sodium 3 mg
Total Carbs 13.1 g
Fiber 1.8 g
Sugar 4.2 g
Protein 0.6 g
Potassium 150 mg

Crème Brûlée

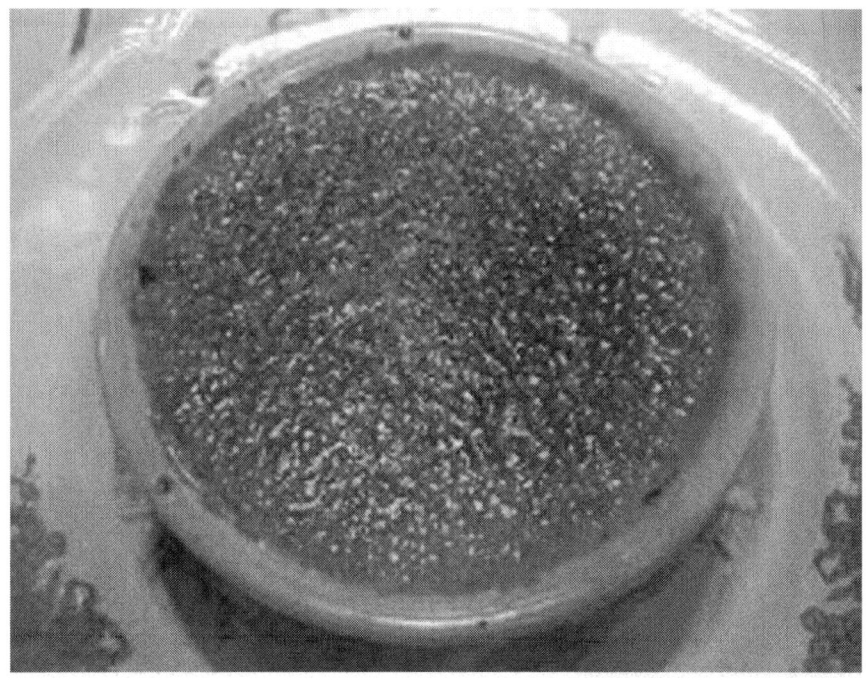

Ingredients:

- ½ teaspoon Splenda
- ½ tablespoon vanilla extract
- 2 egg yolks
- 1 cup heavy cream

How to prepare:
1. Beat together all the ingredients until combined.
2. Divide the mixture evenly in 2 (6-ounce) ramekins.
3. Preheat the oven to 390F and transfer the ramekins in it.

4. Bake for about 13 minutes and transfer the baking dish onto a wire rack to cool for about 30 minutes.
5. Refrigerate the ramekins covered with a plastic wrap for about 3 hours.
6. Serve chilled to the diabetic patients.

Preparation time: 10 minutes
Cooking time: 13 minutes
Total time: 23 minutes
Servings: 2

Nutritional Values:
Calories 289
Total Fat 27.8 g
Saturated Fat 15.9 g
Cholesterol 344 mg
Sodium 33 mg
Total Carbs 3.8 g
Fiber 0 g
Sugar 1.6 g
Protein 4.6 g
Potassium 73 mg

Thai Coconut Custard

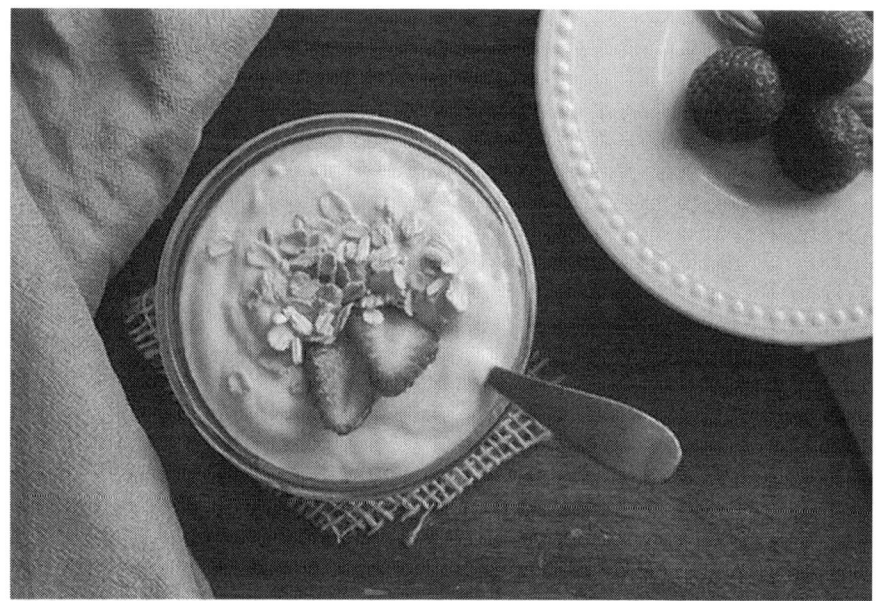

Ingredients:

- 6 eggs
- 2 scoops stevia
- 2 cups unsweetened coconut milk
- 6 drops vanilla extract

How to prepare:
1. Put the coconut milk in a pot and cook on medium-low heat
2. Stir in all the ingredients and cook for about 30 minutes, occasionally stirring.
3. Dish out and serve chilled.

Preparation time: 5 minutes
Cooking time: 30 minutes
Total time: 35 minutes
Servings: 8

Nutritional Values:

Calories 194

Total Fat 17.6 g

Saturated Fat 13.7 g

Cholesterol 123 mg

Sodium 55 mg

Total Carbs 4 g

Fiber 1.3 g

Sugar 2.7 g

Protein 5.5 g

Potassium 207 mg

Chocolate Peanut Butter Cups

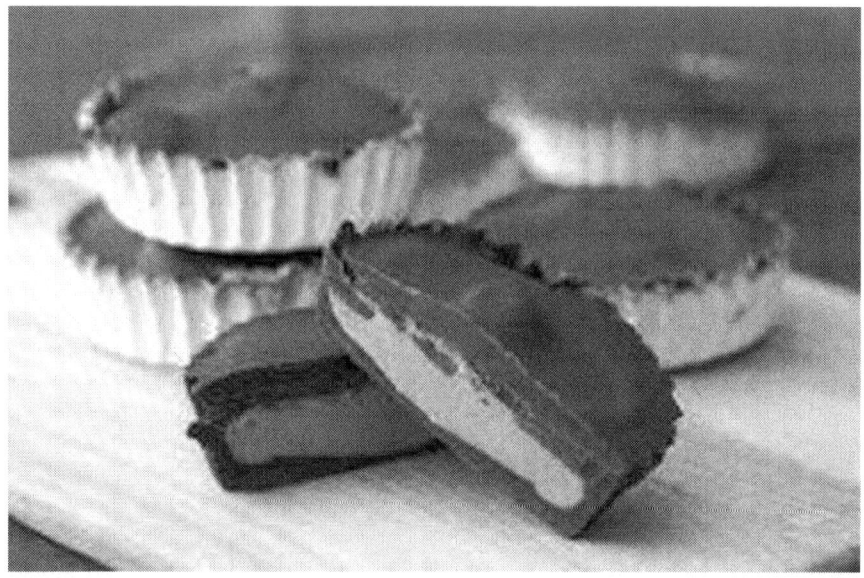

Ingredients:

- 1 ounce unsweetened chocolate
- 2 packets stevia
- 1/8 cup peanut butter, separated
- 1/8 cup heavy cream
- ¼ cup butter

How to prepare:

1. Preheat your oven to 360F and grease the baking mold lightly.

2. Mix together the butter, stevia, unsweetened chocolate, heavy cream, and peanut butter in a bowl.

3. Transfer the mixture in a baking mold and put the baking mold in the oven.

4. Bake for about 30 minutes and dish out.

Preparation time: 15 minutes

Cooking time: 30 minutes

Total time: 45 minutes

Servings: 3

Nutritional Values:

Calories 479

Total Fat 51.5 g

Saturated Fat 29.7 g

Cholesterol 106 mg

Total Carbs 7.7 g

Sugar 1.4 g

Fiber 2.7 g

Sodium 69 mg

Potassium 193 mg

Protein 5.2 g

Cream Crepes

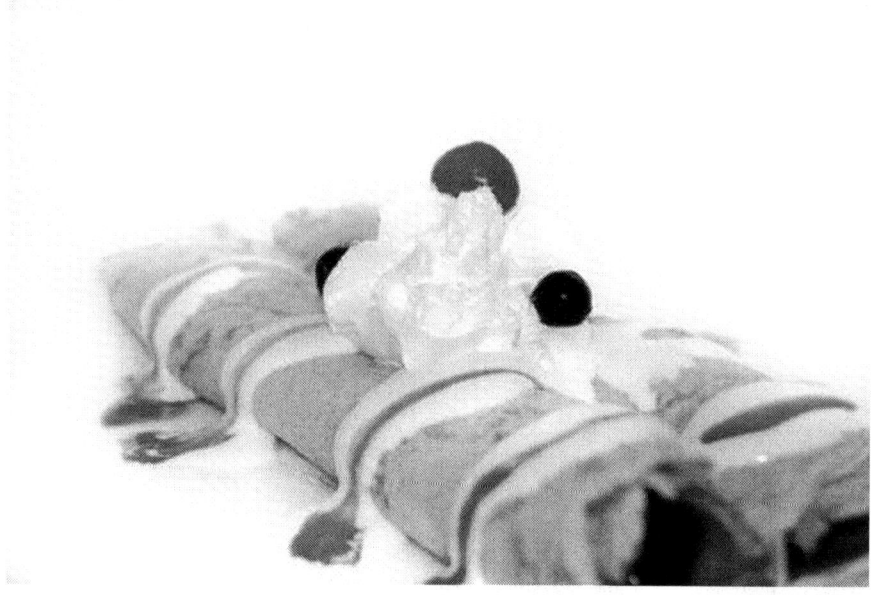

Ingredients:

- 4 organic eggs
- ½ cup heavy cream
- 4 tablespoons coconut flour
- 4 tablespoons olive oil, melted and divided
- 2 scoops stevia

How to prepare:

1. Beat together olive oil, stevia, eggs, and salt in a bowl until well combined.
2. Add the coconut flour slowly and then add the heavy cream while continuously beating.

3. Heat a non-stick pan and pour ¼ of the mixture in it.
4. Cook for about 2 minutes on each side and repeat with the remaining mixture in three batches.

Preparation time: 10 minutes

Cooking time: 16 minutes

Total time: 26 minutes

Servings: 8

Nutritional Values:

Calories 145

Total Fat 13.1 g

Saturated Fat 9.1 g

Cholesterol 96 mg

Total Carbs 4 g

Sugar 1.2 g

Fiber 1.5 g

Sodium 35 mg

Potassium 37 mg

Protein 3.5 g

Nut Porridge

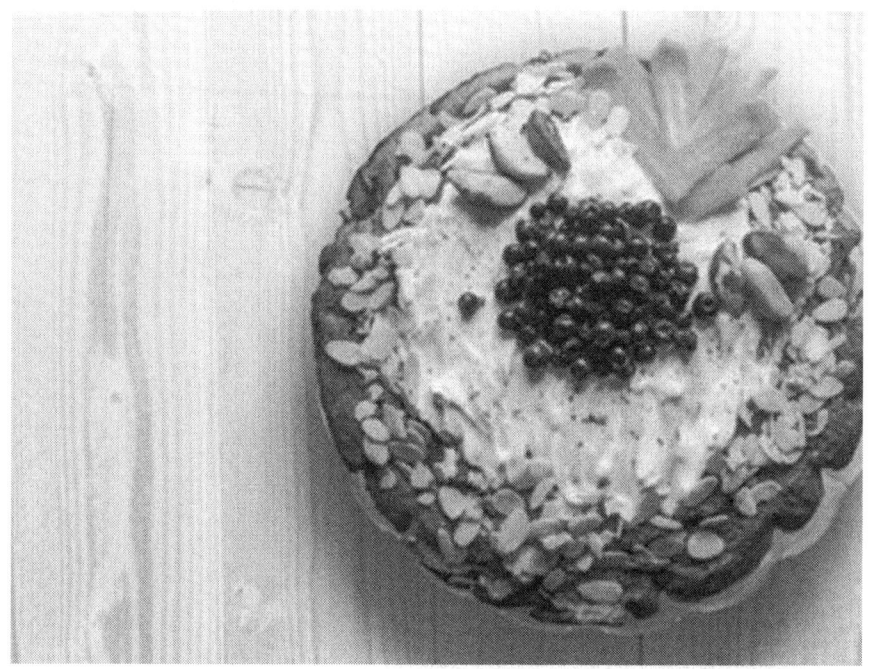

Ingredients:

- 2 cups pecan, halved
- 8 teaspoons coconut oil, melted
- 2 cups cashew nuts, raw and unsalted
- 4 tablespoons stevia
- 4 cups water

How to prepare:
1. Put the pecans and cashew nuts in the food processor and pulse until combined and chunked.
2. Transfer the nuts mixture into the pot and stir in coconut oil, water, and stevia.

3. Simmer on high for 5 minutes and then lower the flame.
4. Simmer on low for 10 minutes and dish out.

Preparation time: 10 minutes
Cooking time: 10 minutes
Total time: 20 minutes
Servings: 8

Nutritional Values:
Calories 260
Total Fat 22.9 g
Saturated Fat 7.3 g
Cholesterol 0 mg
Total Carbs 12.7 g
Sugar 1.8 g
Fiber 1.4 g
Sodium 9 mg
Potassium 209 mg
Protein 5.6 g

BAKERY PRODUCTS RECIPES

Flourless Chocolate Brownies

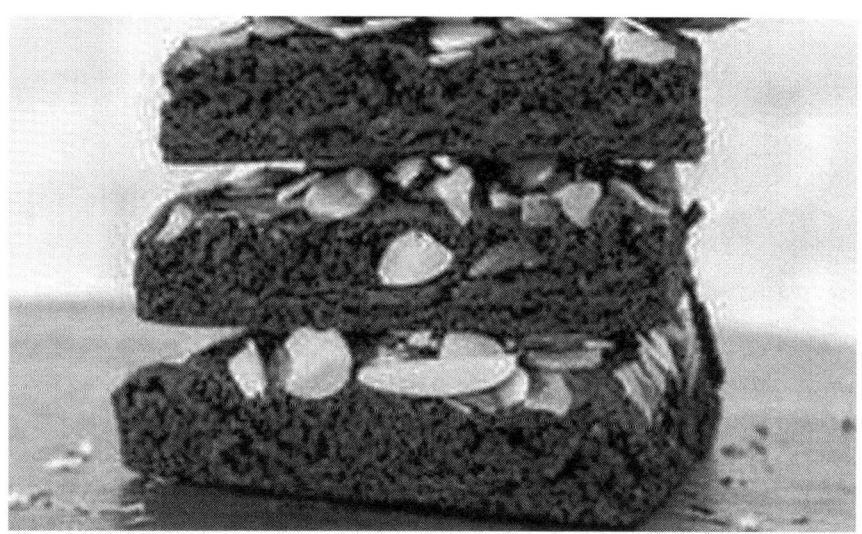

Ingredients:

- 6 eggs
- 2 teaspoons vanilla extract
- 2 packets stevia
- 1 cup butter
- 1 cup sugar-free chocolate chips

How to prepare:
1. Preheat your oven to 395F and grease a baking mold.
2. Whisk together eggs and add stevia and vanilla extract.
3. Put the eggs mixture in the blender and blend until light and frothy.

4. Put the butter and chocolate in a pan and melt on low heat.
5. Add the egg mixture to this melted chocolate mixture.
6. Pour it in the baking mold and transfer the baking mold in the oven.
7. Bake for about 30 minutes and dish out to cut into square pieces to serve.

Preparation time: 10 minutes
Cooking time: 30 minutes
Total time: 40 minutes
Servings: 8

Nutritional Values:
Calories 266
Total Fat 26.9 g
Saturated Fat 15.8 g
Cholesterol 184 mg
Total Carbs 2.5 g
Sugar 0.4 g
Fiber 0 g
Sodium 218 mg
Potassium 53 mg
Protein 4.5 g

Spinach Quiche

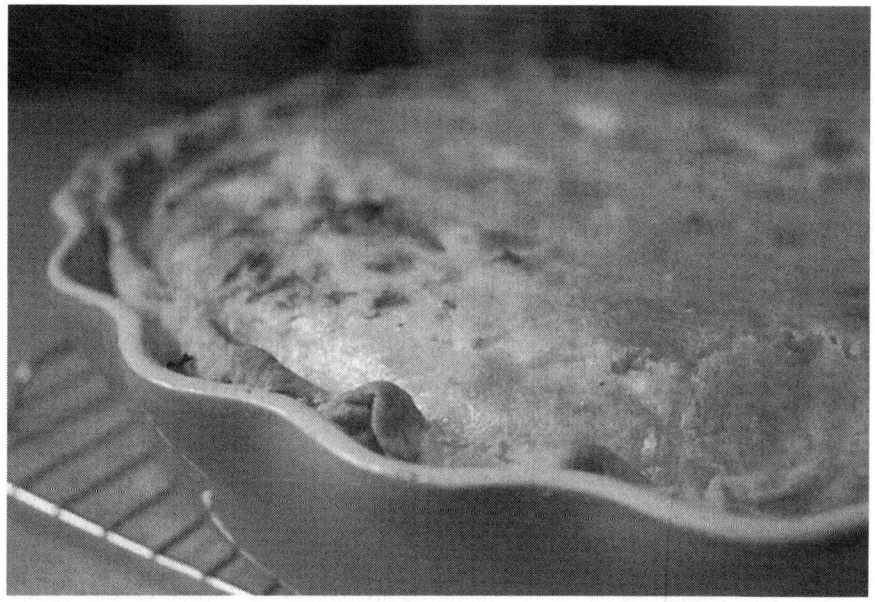

Ingredients:

- 5 organic eggs, beaten
- ½ teaspoon salt and pepper
- 1 (10-ounce) package frozen spinach, thawed
- 1 tablespoon olive oil
- 2 cups Muenster cheese, shredded

How to prepare:
1. Preheat your oven to 350F.
2. Add spinach to heated olive oil in a large skillet.
3. Cook for about 3 minutes and keep aside.
4. Mix together cooked spinach, Muenster cheese, eggs, salt, and black pepper.

5. Transfer the mixture into a greased 9-inch pie dish and bake for about 30 minutes.
6. Cut into wedges to serve.

Preparation time: 10 minutes
Cooking time: 35 minutes
Total time: 45 minutes
Servings: 5

Nutritional Values:

Calories 266

Total Fat 21 g

Saturated Fat 10.4 g

Cholesterol 207 mg

Total Carbs 2.9 g

Sugar 1.1 g

Fiber 1.3 g

Sodium 390 mg

Potassium 436 mg

Protein 17.7 g

Peanut Butter Cookies

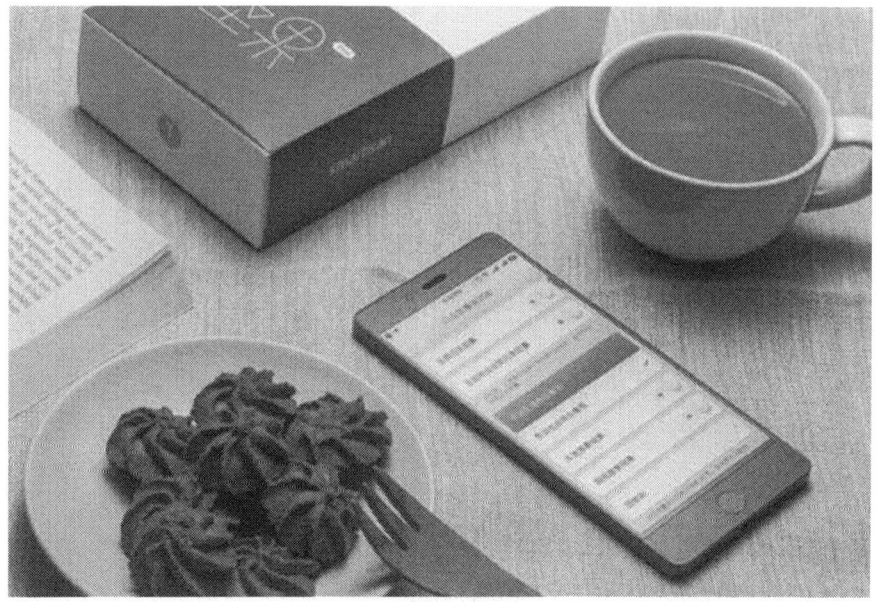

Ingredients:

- 2 teaspoons sugar-free vanilla extract
- 2 scoops stevia
- 2 cups peanut butter
- 1 cup cream
- 2 eggs

How to prepare:
1. Preheat your oven to 360F.
2. Combine cream, peanut butter, egg, stevia, and vanilla extract in a bowl.
3. Mix to form a dough and roll the dough into small balls.

4. Place on the parchment paper lined baking sheet and bake in the preheated oven for 14 minutes.
5. Let cool before serving.

Preparation time: 5 minutes
Cooking time: 15 minutes
Total time: 20 minutes
Servings: 8

Nutritional Values:
Calories 415
Total Fat 35.2 g
Saturated Fat 8.2 g
Cholesterol 47 mg
Total Carbs 14 g
Sugar 6.7 g
Fiber 3.8 g
Sodium 321 mg
Potassium 444 mg
Protein 17.8 g

Cheddar Biscuits

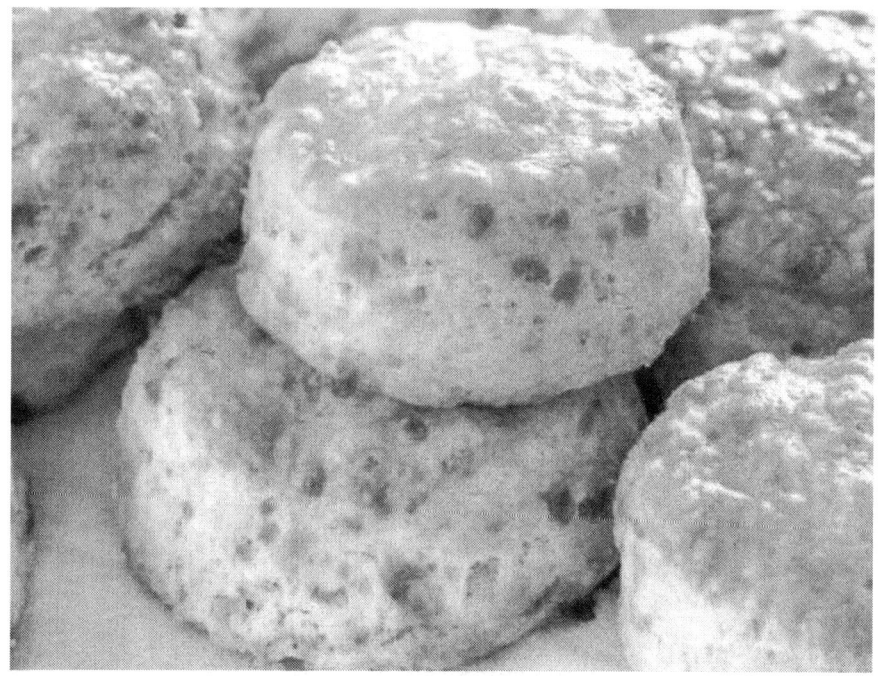

Ingredients:
- 1/8 teaspoon ginger powder
- 1/3 cup coconut flour, sifted
- 2 eggs
- ¼ teaspoon baking powder
- 1/8 cup butter, melted and cooled
- 1/8 teaspoon garlic powder
- ½ cup low-fat sharp cheddar cheese, shredded

How to prepare:
1. Preheat your oven to 400F.
2. Mix together coconut flour, garlic powder, baking powder, and salt in a large bowl.

3. Beat together butter and eggs in another bowl.
4. Mix flour mixture with the egg mixture and beat until well combined.
5. Stir in cheese and transfer the mixture onto foil paper-lined cookie sheets in a single layer.
6. Bake for about 15 minutes and dish out.

Preparation time: 20 minutes
Cooking time: 15 minutes
Total time: 35 minutes
Servings: 4

Nutritional Values:
Calories 180
Total Fat 13.6 g
Saturated Fat 8 g
Cholesterol 112 mg
Sodium 160 mg
Total Carbs 7.3 g
Fiber 4 g
Sugar 0.3 g
Protein 7.7 g
Potassium 78 mg

Cheesecake Cupcakes

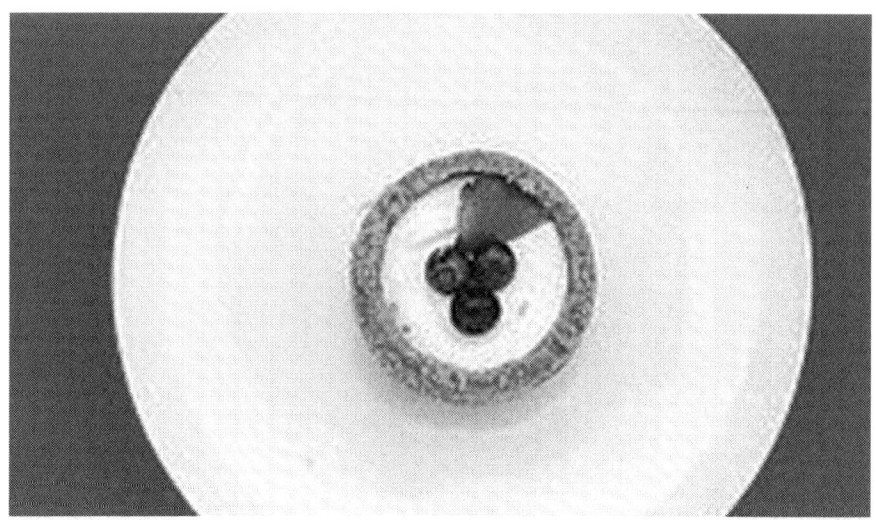

Ingredients:

- 2 (8 ounce) packages cream cheese, softened
- 2 scoops stevia
- 2 eggs
- ½ cup almond meal
- 6 tablespoons butter, melted

How to prepare:

1. Preheat your oven to 350F.
2. Combine almond meal and butter together in a bowl and spoon into the bottom of the paper liners placed in 8 muffin cups and press the mixture into a flat crust.
3. Put cream cheese, eggs, and stevia in a bowl and beat with an electric mixer.

4. Spoon over the crust layer in the paper liners.
5. Bake them 20 minutes and serve.

Preparation time: 10 minutes
Cooking time: 20 minutes
Total time: 30 minutes
Servings: 8

Nutritional Values:

Calories 324

Total Fat 32.5 g

Saturated Fat 18.5 g

Cholesterol 126 mg

Total Carbs 3.1 g

Sugar 0.5 g

Fiber 0.7 g

Sodium 245 mg

Potassium 128 mg

Protein 7 g

Sausage Waffles

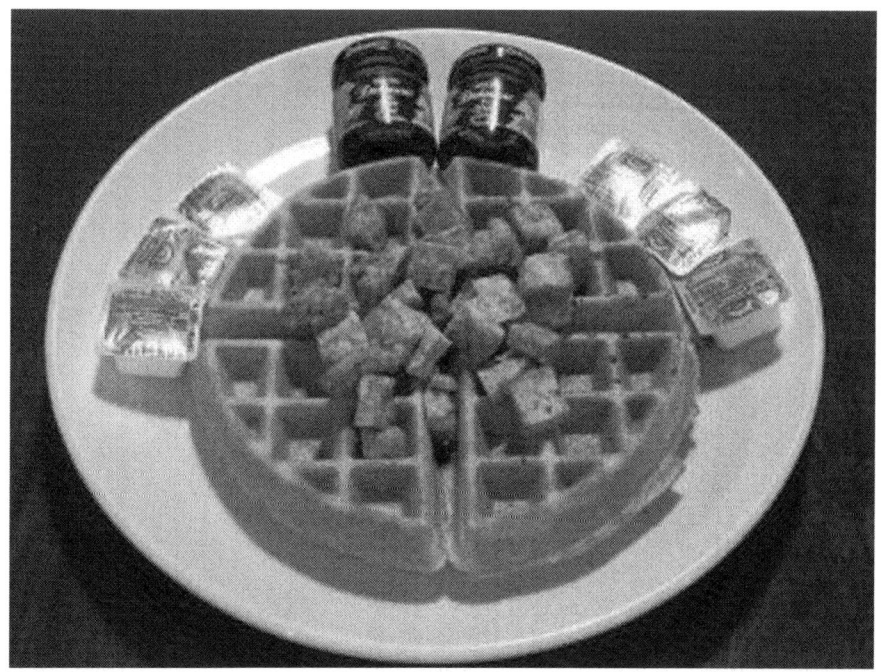

Ingredients:

- 8 medium eggs
- 4 tablespoons red peppers, seeded and chopped
- ½ cup fat-free milk
- 4 tablespoons breakfast sausage, cut into slices
- 4 tablespoons broccoli florets, chopped
- 4 tablespoons low-fat mozzarella cheese, shredded

How to prepare:
1. Preheat a greased waffle iron.
2. Beat together milk and eggs in a bowl and add rest of the ingredients.

3. Stir well and place ¼ of the mixture into preheated waffle iron.
4. Cook for about 5 minutes and repeat with the remaining mixture.

Preparation time: 15 minutes
Cooking time: 20 minutes
Total time: 35 minutes
Servings: 8

Nutritional Values:

Calories 133
Total Fat 8.7 g
Saturated Fat 3.5 g
Cholesterol 177 mg
Sodium 205 mg
Total Carbs 2.2 g
Fiber 0.1 g
Sugar 1.4 g
Protein 11.5 g
Potassium 126 mg

Peach Muffins

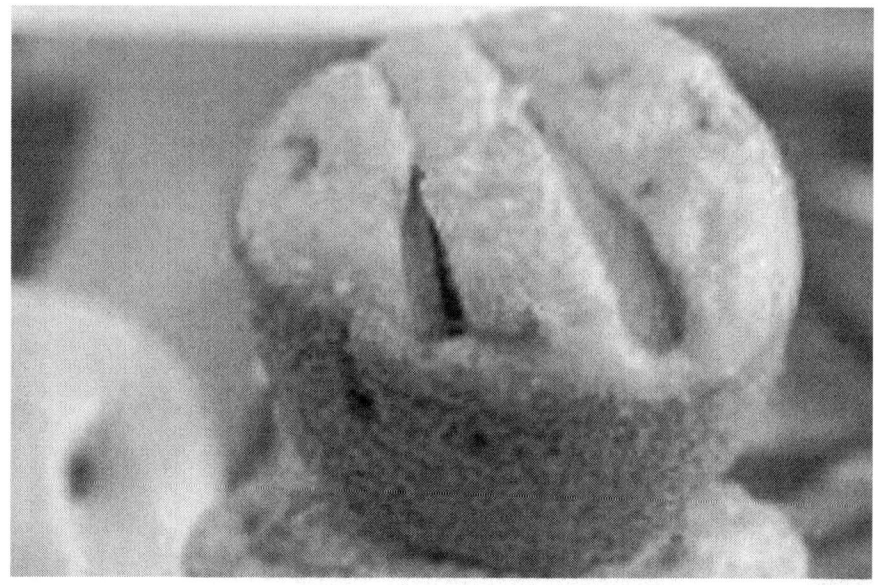

Ingredients:

- ¼ teaspoon baking soda
- 2 eggs
- 1/8 teaspoon vanilla extract
- ½ tablespoon fresh lemon juice
- 1 cup almond flour
- Salt, to taste
- 1 tablespoon butter, melted
- 1 tablespoon unsweetened applesauce
- ½ cup fresh peach, peeled, pitted and chopped finely

How to prepare:

1. Preheat your oven to 325 F.
2. Combine almond flour along with baking soda and salt in a large bowl.
3. Mix together butter, eggs, applesauce, vanilla extract, and lemon juice in another bowl.
4. Beat until well combined and add egg mixture into the flour mixture.
5. Fold in chopped peach and transfer the mixture evenly into 4 greased cups of a large muffin tin.
6. Bake for about 30 minutes and remove the muffin tin from oven.
7. Keep onto a wire rack to cool for about 10 minutes and serve.

Preparation time: 15 minutes

Cooking time: 30 minutes

Total time: 45 minutes

Servings: 4

Nutritional Values:

Calories 235

Total Fat 18.4 g

Saturated Fat 3.5 g

Cholesterol 89 mg

Sodium 180 mg

Total Carbs 8.4 g

Fiber 3.4 g

Sugar 2.4 g

Protein 9 g

Potassium 71 mg

Simple Savory Bread

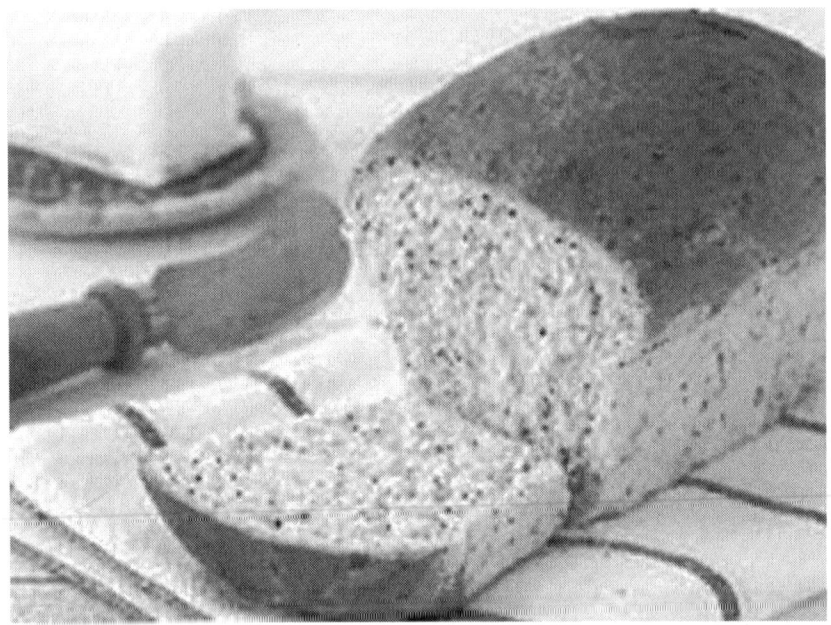

Ingredients:

- ½ teaspoon baking soda
- 1 large egg
- ½ cup almond butter
- ½ tablespoon water
- 1/3 cup almond flour
- ½ teaspoon ground turmeric
- Salt, to taste
- 1 egg white
- ½ tablespoon apple cider vinegar

How to prepare:

1. Preheat your oven to 350F.
2. Mix together flour and baking soda along with turmeric and salt in a large bowl.
3. Mix together eggs, egg whites, water, and cashew butter in another bowl and beat well.
4. Add flour mixture to the eggs mixture and stir in apple cider vinegar.
5. Transfer the mixture evenly into the greased loaf pan and bake for about 20 minutes.
6. Remove the bread pan from oven and keep onto a wire rack to cool for about 10 minutes.
7. Cut the bread loaf in desired sized slices with a sharp knife.

Preparation time: 15 minutes

Cooking time: 20 minutes

Total time: 35 minutes

Servings: 4

Nutritional Values:

Calories 92

Total Fat 6.8 g

Saturated Fat 0.8 g

Cholesterol 47 mg

Sodium 227 mg

Total Carbs 2.7 g

Fiber 1.3 g

Sugar 0.3 g

Protein 4.9 g

Potassium 54 mg

Chocolate Cheese Cake

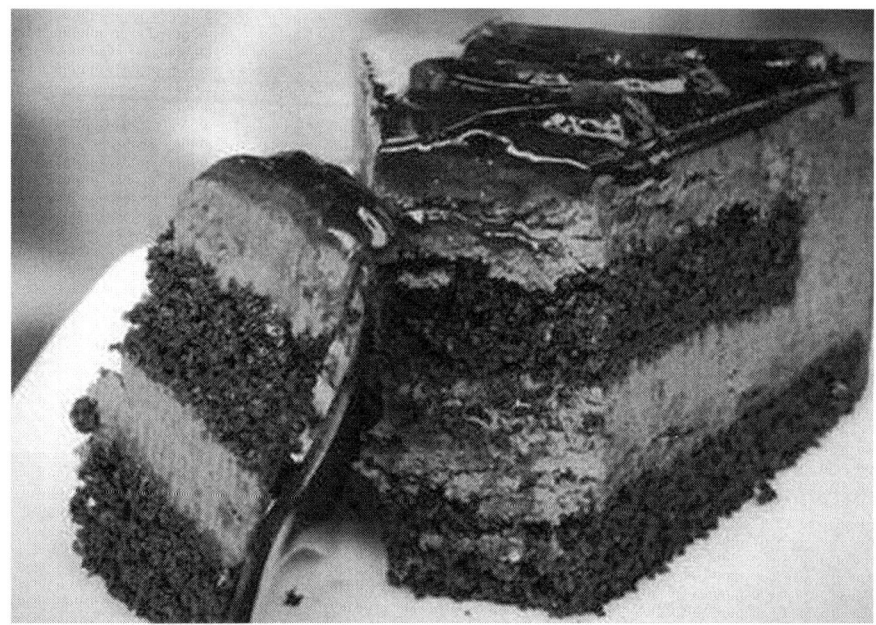

Ingredients:

- 2 eggs
- 1 teaspoon pure vanilla extract
- 2 cups cream cheese, softened
- 2 tablespoons cocoa powder
- 2 scoops stevia

How to prepare:
1. Preheat the oven to 350F.
2. Blend together cream cheese and eggs in a blender until smooth.
3. Pour in the vanilla extract, cocoa powder and stevia and blend again.

4. Add the mixture evenly into 6 (8-ounce) mason jars.
5. Put the mason jars in the oven and bake for about 14 minutes.
6. Chill for 4 hours in a refrigerator before serving.

Preparation time: 10 minutes
Cooking time: 14 minutes
Total time: 24 minutes
Servings: 6

Nutritional Values:

Calories 244

Total Fat 24.8 g

Saturated Fat 15.6 g

Cholesterol 32 mg

Total Carbs 2.1 g

Sugar 0.4 g

Fiber 0.1 g

Sodium 204 mg

Potassium 81 mg

Protein 4 g

21 Days Meal Plan

Week 1

Day 1:
Breakfast: Crustless Mushroom and Bok Choy Quiche
Lunch: Chicken and Mushroom Stew
Dinner: Omega-3 Rich Salmon Soup

Day 2:
Breakfast: Scrambled Eggs with Sausage
Lunch: Cheesy Broccoli Soup
Dinner: Lamb Stew

Day 3:
Breakfast: Cheesy Mini Frittatas
Lunch: Spicy Whole Chicken
Dinner: Egg Soup

Day 4:
Breakfast: Omelet-Topped Rosemary Veggies
Lunch: Asparagus Soup
Dinner: Bright Green Chicken Curry

Day 5:
Breakfast: Asparagus-Cheese Omelet
Lunch: Slow Cooker Mediterranean Stew
Dinner: Chicken and Lime Soup

Day 6:
Breakfast: Spinach Frittata
Lunch: Beef and Veggies Soup
Dinner: Air Fried Chicken

Day 7:
Breakfast: Onion Tofu Scramble
Lunch: Salmon Stew
Dinner: Ground Beef Soup

Week2

Day 1:
Breakfast: Sausage Solo
Lunch: Paprika Shrimp
Dinner: Salmon Soup

Day 2:
Breakfast: Sausage Bacon Beans Cancan
Lunch: Shrimp Soup
Dinner: Special Butter Fish

Day 3:
Breakfast: Eggs Stuffed with Avocado and Watercress
Lunch: Harvested Chicken Stew
Dinner: Omega-3 Rich Salmon Soup

Day 4:
Breakfast: Crustless Mushroom and Bok Choy Quiche
Lunch: Cheesy Broccoli Soup
Dinner: Shrimp Curry

Day 5:
Breakfast: Scrambled Eggs with Sausage
Lunch: Egg Soup
Dinner: Mexican Beef Brisket

Day 6:
Breakfast: Cheesy Mini Frittatas
Lunch: Asparagus Soup
Dinner: Citrus Glazed Salmon

Day 7:
Breakfast: Omelet-Topped Rosemary Veggies
Lunch: Chicken and Lime Soup
Dinner: Beef Bulgogi

Week 3

Day 1:
Breakfast: Asparagus-Cheese Omelet
Lunch: Beef and Veggies Soup
Dinner: Delicious Lobster

Day 2:
Breakfast: Spinach Frittata
Lunch: Salmon Soup
Dinner: Cheesy Cauliflower

Day 3:
Breakfast: Onion Tofu Scramble
Lunch: Ground Beef Soup
Dinner: Jamaican Jerk Pork Roast

Day 4:
Breakfast: Sausage Solo
Lunch: Shrimp Soup
Dinner: Pork Carnitas

Day 5:
Breakfast: Sausage Bacon Beans Cancan
Lunch: Slow Cooker Mediterranean Stew
Dinner: Asparagus Soup

Day 6:
Breakfast: Eggs Stuffed with Avocado and Watercress
Lunch: Salmon Soup
Dinner: Mexican Beef Brisket

Day 7:
Breakfast: Cheesy Mini Frittatas
Lunch: Lamb Stew
Dinner: Egg Soup

CONCLUSION:

Type 2 diabetes is a medical condition in which the blood sugar levels (glucose) rises above the allowed limit or its normal value. It is also known as 'hyperglycemia.' It is also referred to as a long term metabolic disorder in which there is lack of insulin, higher blood sugar levels, and insulin resistance. It can be easily lived with an anti-diabetic life style supported by medications.

Legal Notice

This document is geared towards providing exact and reliable information in regards to the topic and issue covered. The publication is sold with the idea that the publisher is not required to render accounting, officially permitted, or otherwise, qualified services. If advice is necessary, legal or professional, a practiced individual in the profession should be ordered.

From a Declaration of Principles which was accepted and approved equally by a Committee of the American Bar Association and a Committee of Publishers and Associations.

In no way is it legal to reproduce, duplicate, or transmit any part of this document in either electronic means or in printed format. Recording of this publication is strictly prohibited and any storage of this document is not allowed unless with written permission from the publisher. All rights reserved.

The information provided herein is stated to be truthful and consistent, in that any liability, in terms of inattention or otherwise, by any usage or abuse of any policies, processes, or directions contained within is the solitary and utter responsibility of the recipient reader. Under no circumstances will any legal responsibility or blame be held against the publisher for any reparation, damages, or monetary loss due to the information herein, either directly or indirectly.

Respective authors own all copyrights not held by the publisher.

The information herein is offered for informational purposes solely, and is universal as so. The presentation of the information is without contract or any type of guarantee assurance.

The trademarks that are used are without any consent, and the publication of the trademark is without permission or backing by the trademark owner. All trademarks and brands within this book are for clarifying purposes only and are owned by the owners themselves, not affiliated with this document.

Printed in Great Britain
by Amazon